OPIATE ADDICTION, MORALITY AND MEDICINE

Opiate Addiction, Morality and Medicine

From Moral Illness to Pathological Disease

Geoffrey Harding

Researcher, Department of Pharmaceutics
School of Pharmacy, University of London

St. Martin's Press New York

Scholarly & Reference Division,
St. Martin's Press, Inc., 175 Fifth Avenue, New York, NY 10010

First published in the United States of America in 1988

Printed in Hong Kong

ISBN 0–312–01201–2

Library of Congress Cataloging-in-Publication Data
Harding, Geoffrey, 1954–
Opiate addiction, morality, and medicine.
Includes bibliographies and index.
1. Narcotic habit—Great Britain—History.
2. Narcotic habit—Great Britain—Moral and ethical aspects—History. 3. Opium habit—Great Britain—History. I. Title. [DNLM: 1. Narcotic Dependence—history—Great Britain. 2. Opium—history—Great Britain. WM 11 H263o]
HV 5840.G7H34 1988 362.2'93 87–13138
ISBN 0–312–01201–2

To Dave and Mary

Contents

Acknowledgements

My thanks are due to the Economic and Social Research Council, which funded the research for the thesis on which this book is based. I am also grateful for the guidance and encouragement of Gerry Stimson, who acted as my supervisor. Particular thanks are due to Martin Clarke, who made valuable constructive criticisms, provided unstinting support and diligently checked earlier drafts with enduring patience and goodwill.

GEOFFREY HARDING

Introduction

In Great Britain during the first half of the nineteenth century addiction to opium was regarded at worst as a minor vice – in many respects akin to today's heavy smoker or drinker. In 1840, in a prominent medical journal of the day a physician, Dr Thompson, was moved to record his view that opium, when taken as a stimulant, i.e. not for any recognisable medical complaint but merely as a cheap alternative to drink, 'acted as an aphrodisiac and subverted all morality' and added that it 'affected all that was good and virtuous in women'.[1]

Towards the end of the century this popular idea of addiction as mere bad habit was challenged by a growing number of physicians who deemed it to be a sickness – a diseased state which required medical treatment. In 1878 in Britain, one prescribed treatment for morphia addicts was abrupt withdrawal ('cold turkey' in American parlance, describing the gooseflesh appearance of the addict's skin accompanying withdrawal). Attended by nurses and overseen by a physician, the addict's supply of morphia would be abruptly withdrawn, to be replaced, during the most difficult period of withdrawal pains by recourse to warm baths, bicarbonate of soda, chloral hydrate and unlimited amounts of champagne and brandy![12]

Just under fifty years later, in 1926, the Home Office endorsed the recommendations of a Committee chaired by Sir Humphrey Rolleston, late president of the Royal College of Physicians of London and Regius Professor of Physics at Cambridge, that addicts could legally receive treatment from a physician which involved being given a regular prescription for a measured amount of an opiate. Depending on the particular case the dosage might be gradually reduced but could be maintained indefinitely, depending on the judgement of the attending physician. In the course of a relatively short time then, it was possible for drug addiction to be spoken of as a mere bad habit or at worse a vice, and latterly as a medically treatable sickness.

The history of responses to addiction does not begin with the first addicts. Opium had already been used in England and other European countries for several centuries and addiction undoubtedly featured in many a lifestyle. Instead it begins with the first *responses* to drug use. But the development of these responses is puzzling. How was it possible for people to talk of opium dependence in certain ways, for example as a vice; and how was it possible for a new understanding of opium dependence as a medically defined disease, to emerge from a previous, widely subscribed understanding of addiction as an issue of immorality? These themes are dealt with in subsequent chapters. First though, no discussion on the social responses to opiate addiction would be adequate without some broad understanding of the history of its use and of its psycho-pharmacological effects on the user.

Papaver Somniferum

Opium, the base drug from which opiates are extracted, is obtained from the white poppy, *Papaver Somniferum*. The poppy's seed capsule is incised just after the petals have fallen but before it is fully ripe, using a sharp multibladed knife known amongst Indian cultivators as a *nashtar* or *nurnee*. From the incision exudes a milky juice which dries on contact with the air to form a brownish gummy mass. Extracting the opium is a skilful task; if the incision is too shallow no juice is exuded, too deep an incision and the juice flows inwards and is lost among the seeds. By-products of *Papaver Somniferum* include its seeds which are used in cooking or pressed for their oil, and the petals which were once regarded as imperative in processing the drug for export.

The poppy was first discovered in the Eastern Mediterranean and its effects were known to the Sumerians 6000 years ago. Galen, a Roman physician of the second century A.D., was an enthusiastic advocate of the poppy, and his teachings remained authoritative for centuries. Following the decline of the Roman Empire, the use of opium spread to the Middle East where Arab physicians became well versed in its applications. Arab traders introduced the drug to the Far East where it was used, until the seventeenth century, mainly to control dysentery.

In the following century, as tobacco smoking spread through Europe to the Orient, the smoking of opium, mixed with tobacco but latterly on its own, became increasingly popular in China despite attempts by Chinese authorities to eradicate this practice. The Chinese even developed a special pipe for the purpose of smoking opium. Lieutenant Bingham, a British Naval Officer, described a pipe he purchased as a souvenir in Canton as being seventeen inches long, one inch in diameter with a turned mouthpiece made from buffalo's horn. The bowl, three inches in diameter with a pin-sized puncture on its upper side, was made from clay and resembled the shape of a 'flattened turnip'. Unlike tobacco, the smoking of opium involves a laborious preparatory process. A drop of opium gum is first placed on the point of a needle and heated over a flame where it gradually turns pale, softens, swells and begins to bubble and splutter. It is then quickly carried to the surface of the pipe's bowl, before it turns to vapour, and the bowl is then tipped into an open flame. The heavy white smoke that results is then inhaled. Two or three puffs and the drop is consumed and the process may have to be repeated several times until the effects are felt.

PSYCHO-PHARMACOLOGICAL EFFECTS OF OPIATES

The pharmacological action of opiates produces a number of physiological effects. The short-term effects include a reduction in cardio-vascular activity, contraction of the pupils, a minor reduction in visual acuity, a dilation of the cutaneous blood vessels and a slight itching.[3] On the central nervous system opiates produce a selective analgesic effect. They rapidly reduce levels of pain, most effectively for dull continuous rather than sharp intermittent attacks. As the dose is increased the other subjective effects of mood alteration and mental clouding – which are characterised by drowsiness, inability to concentrate, apathy, lessening of physical activity and lethargy – become more pronounced. When small to moderate amounts of an opiate are given to patients with pain, discomfort, worry or tension, the pain is reported to be less intense and therefore less distressing, if indeed it has not entirely gone.[4] In addition to the relief of distressing pain, some patients were observed to experience euphoria. However, when opiates are administered in the same dosage to pain-free individuals the experience was not always as pleasant, often with dysphoria marked by mild anxiety or fear and frequent nausea with occasional vomiting.

Opiates can produce respiratory depression with all but the smallest doses. They also depress the cough reflex and this makes them therapeutically useful particularly in controlling non-productive, exhausting coughs. The other major effects of opiates are on the gastro-intestinal tract, where they are readily absorbed into the gut. By diminishing the propulsive peristaltic waves in the intestinal tract, the action of the opiate combines to produce a constipating effect on the bowel.

Regular administration of opiates produces a change in physiological reactivity. This change is manifested by the development of physical dependence and tolerance to opiates. Physical dependence is exhibited by the symptoms of abstinence or 'withdrawal syndrome', following termination of the drug. Yawning, perspiration, gooseflesh, dilated pupils, restlessness, sexual orgasm, increased blood pressure, vomiting, diarrhoea and insomnia are among the most prominent symptoms. Tolerance is manifested by a diminution in the physiological effects of opiates and is most rapidly acquired for opiate's euphoric effect and relatively slowly gained for the analgesic effect.

The therapeutic effects of opium derive from natural alkaloids contained in the opium poppy. Well over twenty alkaloids have been identified and they constitute 25 per cent of opium's weight. The first alkaloid to be discovered was morphine – named after Morpheus, the Greek god of dreams – by Serturner, a German apothecary, in 1803. Subsequent alkaloids discovered include Codeine, in 1848, and the less popularly familiar substances thebane, papaverine and noscapine. Diacetylmorphine or diamorphine – a semi-synthetic derivative of morphine made by simple modification of morphine's original chemical structure – was discovered at St Mary's Hospital, London, in 1874. However, it was not introduced into medical practice until 1891 by the Bayer Company of Germany who marketed it as a remedy for coughs, under the trade name Heroin.

OPIUM: THE UNIVERSAL PANACEA

In the nineteenth century opium was the most widely used drug of its day, very much like aspirin is today. It was rarely smoked and, until the nineteenth century, was consumed in its raw state in various forms. Cut from a solid block the crude opium would be shaped into pills for sale from pharmacies or sold in square blocks by general grocers. By the nineteenth century a variety of preparations which contained opium, developed in Europe had become available in Britain, the most popular being laudanum or tincture of opium. This was first compounded by Paracelsus at Basle, in the fifteenth century, by mixing raw opium with distilled water and alcohol. The seventeenth-century physician, Thomas Sydenham, was an enthusiastic prescriber of laudanum and was given to extol the virtues of its active ingredient, opium, thus,

> Among the remedies which it has pleased Almighty God to give to man to relieve his suffering, none is so universal and so efficacious as opium.[5] . . . This medicine is so necessary an instrument in the hands of a skilful person, that the art of medicine would be imperfect without it, and whoever is thoroughly acquainted with its virtues, and the manner of using it, will perform greater things than might reasonably be expected from the use of any single medicine.[6]

In the eighteenth century Le Mort, Professor of Chemistry at the University of Leyden, combined opium with camphor to produce paragoric which proved an effective control for diarrhoea.

1 Opium and the British

In 1753, George Young wrote in the preface to his *Treatise on Opium* that, 'opium has already got into the hands of every pretender to practice, and is prescribed every day, not only by the many charitable and well-meaning ladies, but by the too officious and ignorant nurses', and added that he found opium to be a 'slow poison'.[1] None the less until the mid-nineteenth century, opium and an array of various opium containing preparations could be bought, sold and consumed, without concern. Opium, which was freely imported into Britain, was also a lucrative trade for the wholesale druggists who saw the import duty payable on it drop from four shillings a pound weight in 1828 to one shilling a pound weight in 1836, and finally abolished in 1860.[2] Commensurately, levels of imported opium rose from 17 000lb in 1827, equal to 600mg per head, per year, to 35 000lb in 1833; and during the 1850s reached upwards of 55 000lb a year. By 1859, consumption had risen to 61 000lb per year, equivalent to an individual daily dose of 1410mg.[3]

Opium and opium-based preparations were cheap – with raw opium selling for sixpence an ounce and an average daily dose of 30 grams costing only a penny. They were also readily available from a number of retail outlets, the most popular of these being chemists, apothecaries and general dealers. These were, however, by no means the exclusive retailers of opium. In 1865, those selling drugs in the market town of Preston included: 'a basket maker, shoe maker, small-ware dealer, factory operative, tailor, rubbing stone maker and baker, a rent collector who . . . was connected with the buryin' trade'.[4] It was even sold on market stalls and by itinerant hawkers.

A bewildering range of commercial preparations were also sold. One manufacturer of such preparations, George Meggeson, included in his price list opium lozenges made with opium, opium and chalk, opium and fruit, morphia, morphia and ipecacuanha, poppy, and paregoric. Opium syrups and pills were another variation, made from opium and soap, or opium and lead. But the more popular commercial preparations included Dover's powders – a mixture of ipecacuanha and powdered opium and Collis Brown's

Chlorodyne. Specific opium-based preparations were developed for consumption by children – children's draughts with such promising names as Godfrey's Cordial, Dalby's Carminative, Pennyworth of Peace and Daffy's Elixir.[5] In addition to these commercial preparations there was a beverage called poppy tea – which was made in the home, from the poppy head – a well-known remedy for soothing fractious babies.

Raw opium, sold in penny-worths, was bought as a cheap and freely available curative for use in medical practice or self-medication by a population which had little access to constant medical care. In the belief that it was a universal panacea, opium was taken for such trivial complaints as earache or influenza as much as for the more serious ones such as hydrophobia, haemorrhage and heart disease.[6] Jonathan Pereira included opium in his well-known text, *Elements of Materia Medica*, claiming, 'opium is undoubtedly the most important and valuable remedy of the whole Materia Medica. We have, for all the medicines one or more substitutes; for opium we have none' and he recommended its use, 'to mitigate pain, to ally spasms, to promote sleep, to reduce nervous restlessness, to produce perspiration; and to check profuse mucous discharge from the bronchial tube and gastro-intestinal canal'.[7] It was bought most popularly by the working class factory operatives as a remedy for fatigue and depression – a presumably unavoidable condition in a life characterised by strenuous labour, poverty and hunger – their dependence on opium often going unnoticed until their supply was curtailed.

In the 1850s, it was conservatively estimated that in England there were between 16 000 and 25 000 outlets for the sale of opium.[8] Acceptance of opium was such as to encourage experimentation by enterprising farmers, doctors and gardeners with domestic cultivation of the opium poppy. Attempts to grow British opium date back to the 1740s[9] and continued on a piecemeal basis until the 1870s[10] but interest peaked during the years 1790 to 1820. (In 1830 an Edinburgh man succeeded in getting 56lbs of raw opium from one acre of the plant.) It was the Society of Arts which first actively encouraged extensive experimentation of domestic cultivation of opium. Awards of fifty guineas or a gold medal were offered to those who produced at least twenty pounds of domestically cultivated raw opium. By 1810, the Caledonian Horticultural Society was offering medals for the most efficient method for cultivating the plant in British soil. But despite glowing testimonies as to the efficacy and purity of the British opium, and owing to the vagaries of the British climate, the comparative ease of growing alternative crops, and the relatively cheap cost of agricultural labour abroad, domestic cultivation of opium was never commercially successful.

The use of opium imported into Britain continued along with an essentially relaxed attitude to its consumption for much of the early nineteenth century. Acceptance of the non-medical use of opium is illustrated in the response (or rather the lack of response) evoked by confessions of opium eating among the literary middle classes. Thomas De Quincey is perhaps the most celebrated example and his work has become a milestone in the history of opium in Britain. De Quincey began taking opium at regular intervals in 1804, principally as a remedy for gastric pains. Indeed, in a letter to Wordsworth in 1809, he was given to lament the bad effects of 'accidently' swallowing some opium he was holding in his mouth for a toothache. By 1814, however, his repeated use of the drug had left him dependent on it. Writing to a friend, Crabb Robinson in 1816, De Quincey explained their meeting would have to take place in the afternoon because opium kept him from rising in the morning. The sensationalist title of De Quincey's most famous work, *Confessions of an English Opium Eater*, is however misleading. The idea of the 'Confessions' was possibly borrowed from his friend, Charles Lamb who wrote *Confessions of a Drunkard* in 1813. Following publication of De Quincey's work there subsequently emerged a spate of similar 'Confessions': James Hogg's *Confessions of a Justified Sinner* (1824); Countess of Blessington's *Confessions of an Inquiring Spirit* (1840); Thackeray's *The Confessions of Fitz-Boodle* (1852); which were all possibly influenced by De Quincey's earlier example.

De Quincey's *Confessions* first appeared anonymously in 1821 in two instalments of *The London Magazine* under the title *Confessions of an English Opium Eater: Being an Extract from the Life of a Scholar*. They were based on an autobiographical framework which cobbled together some already written prose describing his opium dreams. But their publication in book form the following year were not 'confessions' in the true sense of the word as they contained no sense of remorse. 'Guilt', De Quincey wrote, 'I do not acknowledge'. If anything, the book, in its earlier versions, celebrated his triumph in overcoming opium dependency, though somewhat prematurely for in later life he went through three more periods of attempting to give up opium. Indeed, before he died he was still taking opium, albeit in moderate doses, despite contending that his application of will-power and courage had helped him resist, 'the seduction of opium to the final extremity', and had shown that the 'deep bondage' might be cut off.

Earlier editions indeed issued caution to would-be users of opium but De Quincey's work was not written as an exposé to warn an unsuspecting public of the dangers surrounding its use. In the final version he lauded opium's 'beneficial characteristics' which he believed had prevented him from contracting tuberculosis – the disease from which his father had died. Moreover, the stuporific effects of opium, he maintained, were eminently preferable to those which followed alcohol intoxication. 'The opium eater . . . feels that the divine part of his nature is paramount – that is, the moral affections are in a state of cloudless serenity; and high overall the great light of the majestic intellect.'[11]

It is this notion of a 'majestic intellect' which provided the principle theme of the *Confessions*. 'I was necessarily ignorant of the whole art and mystery of opium taking; and what I took, I took under every disadvantage. But I took it: and in an hour, oh! heavens! what a revelation! what an unheaving, from its lowest depths, of the inner spirit! what an apocalypse of the world within me! That my pain had vanished, was now a trifle in my eyes: this negative effect was swallowed up in the immensity of those positive effects which had opened before me – in the abyss of divine enjoyment thus suddenly revealed.'[12]

Well over a century later the notion of an opium-induced 'majestic intellect' or 'romantic imagination' continued to be debated. Elizabeth Schnider's[13] study of the famous opium-eating poet Coleridge, concluded emphatically that the drug had no constructive effect on the abilities of the writers and poets. More recently Hayter[14] in a similar study concludes otherwise. Although opium was initially taken by the likes of De Quincey and Coleridge for medicinal reasons its use shaded into social or 'stimulant' usage and Hayter points to Coleridge's Kubla Khan, which, she maintains, was produced under the influence of opium. But it was De Quincey's *Confessions of an Opium Eater*, first published in book form in 1822, which provided the first detailed account of English opium eating and its effects on the creative imagination. Reaction to the first publication of *'Confessions'* evoked a blend of curiosity – possible because the majority of descriptions available had portrayed the habit, especially of opium smoking, as a peculiarly Eastern custom – with a sense of moral indignation.

This air of calm interest in the effects of opium on literary creations carried through to the mid-nineteenth century. Wilkie Collins, who regularly consumed laudanum by the glassful – a large dose by comparison, saw nothing wrong in introducing it into his immensely popular novel *The Moonstone*. An unsurprising move in an era in which the attitude to opium was one of tolerance. Temperate use hardly gave rise to comment, let along concern, and discussions of opium's effects focused on its therapeutic rather than its harmful effects. Excessive use by the working class had yet to become a major issue of concern and was ignored by all but a few public health campaigners, while similar use among the middle classes was regarded as a minor vice. Amidst this liberal attitude in which opium taking was regarded a matter for the individual, the development of an initial response to the non-medical use of opium was therefore not concerned with whether it was consumed merely as a stimulant or not. Such expressions of moralistic concern were barely audible. What originally was at issue was the effects, if any, the non-medical use of opium had on life expectancy.

THE CASE OF THE EARL OF MAR

The issue first came to prominence following the death of the Earl of Mar in 1928. The Earl died of jaundice and dropsy, having first taken out several insurance policies on his life. Following submission of a claim by his executors an investigation by the insurance companies revealed that the Earl had been in the habit of taking laudanum 'to excess' and the insurance companies refused to pay out. The issue was subsequently taken up in court where the insurance companies argued that opium eating was a habit which affected health and longevity and therefore should have been stated when first taking out the policies. However the court ruled against them on the grounds that they had shown insufficient care when conducting their preliminary enquiries into the Earl's habit.

Subsequent medical interest in the case led Robert Christison, Professor of Medical Jurisprudence at Edinburgh University, to judge – on the basis of his own personal survey of opium eaters –

that opium and its sustained use did not produce any physically damaging condition.[15]

What was at issue in the medical discussions following the Earl of Mar case was the possible effects and consequences of opium consumption. The notion of opium habituation itself was not a medical concern. If anything, it was a moral issue, though condemnation of the non-medical use of opium was scarcely evident until mid-century. Although it was wrong to drink laudanum as De Quincey had – purportedly to stimulate a romantic imagination – it was right to take opium for toothache.[16]

OPIUM: AN EMERGENT PROBLEM

When opium was introduced into Britain in the seventeenth century it was exalted as a universal panacea for all ills. Its widespread acceptance as an invaluable curative remained unchallenged for approximately two hundred years. By the second half of the nineteenth century however, official moves were afoot which ultimately led to the drawing up of legislative measures to control the availablity and consumption of opium. The longevity debate was certainly significant in drawing medical attention to the effects of its use. Indeed it represented the first development in medical thinking on the effects of opium and was to mark the beginning of a more extensive medical involvement in the question of opium use. But the development of a response directed towards controlling the use of opium – in the second half of the nineteenth century – did not result directly from medical testimonies which denounced the effects resulting from its sustained consumption. So why did this change in attitude towards drugs and the way in which they were perceived occur?

Berridge and Edwards[17] have taken up this issue in their account of nineteenth-century opium use in Great Britain. Setting the popular use of opium in the wider social context of late Victorian society, they point to the growing concern over British involvement in the trade in opium, and agitation by the temperance movement, as significant developments in the changing attitude towards widespread use of opium. Underscoring their thesis is the argument that the British response to opiate use during the last century was developed as a scapegoat for wider class-based tensions which featured prominently during the developing stages of British industrialisation. The concept of opium use as an issue of concern was created from within the class tensions of two mid-nineteenth-century developments – the emergence of a public health cause, and the development of separate pharmaceutical and medical professions. In each it was not the inherent dangers of opium for an unsuspecting public that was at stake but the opportunity for these professions to develop a system of domination over the lower classes.

Until the first half of the nineteenth century, they argue, the consumption of opium existed primarily as a working class, culturally sanctioned practice which was restricted largely to self-medication. But this practice provoked a distinct mid-century reaction which culminated in opium being allocated a minor part in the public health cause. It first emerged as an issue in the public health campaign against the adulteration of drugs. Evidence of deaths attributed to accidental overdoses of opium was revealed in the poisoning statistics that were beginning to be compiled around the middle of the nineteenth century and this, Berridge and Edwards suggest, pointed to the need for some form of regulation or control over the drug's supply.

The mid-century public health campaign focused its enquiries almost exclusively on the working class's culturally regulated use of opium. One aspect of their use of the drug which recurred in reports following the campaign's enquiries concerned the practice by some working mothers of doping their infants with opium in order to soothe them before leaving them in the charge of old women or very young girls. The 1844-45 Commission on the State of Large Towns drew attention to the fact that in Preston over 1600 families were in the habit of using 'Godfrey's' regularly. Engels's investigations into the conditions of the working class in Manchester also emphasised this aspect of opium consumption. A druggist working in the city was recorded to have sold upwards of five gallons of his own brand of 'Quietness' – a preparation for soothing fractious babies – containing one hundred drops of laudanum to the ounce, supplying seven hundred households a week. Another druggist in the Lancashire town of Thorpe was reported to have sold a gallon of laudanum and two to three pounds of opium at market in one day. One nineteenth-century commentator observed that 'On market days, they come in from Lynn and Warrington and buy the pure drug for themselves, and Godfrey's' or 'Quietness' for their children.'[18]

When these practices came to the attention of public health campaigners there followed the claim that working mothers were the root cause of infant doping. Such exaggerated claims, Berridge and Edwards argue, exhibit a complete insensitivity to the cultural and economic life of the Victorian working class. Most mothers with young children, they suggest, did not in fact work. This in turn, however led to a lower standard of nutrition for the babies due to the family's being economically worse off. The campaign's enquiries also showed a total disregard for any beneficial effects which working-class culture believed infant dosing with opium might have – for instance in easing the child's digestive complaints cause by poor nutrition. Moreover, these criticisms of infant doping served to divert attention from the inequities of nineteenth-century working-class life and focus it on the individual failings of working-class mothers.

Concern with infant dosing also lead to enquiries over adult working-class consumption. Attention to the possibility of 'stimulant' or recreational use of opium among the urban poor was first drawn by publication of De Quincey's *Confessions*. In it he described what was later to form the popular view of working-class opium use – taken as a 'dram' – and a cheaper alternative to alcohol:

> Some years ago, in passing through Manchester, I was informed by several cotton manufacturers that their work people were rapidly getting into the practice of opium eating; so much so that on a Saturday afternoon the counters of the druggist were strewn with pills of one, two or three grains, in preparations for the known demand of the evening. The immediate occasion of this practice was the lowness of wages at that time would not allow them to indulge in ale and spirit.[19]

Indeed opium and its preparations were widely consumed in a number of other industrial towns and cities, including Sheffield, Birmingham and Nottingham, as self-prescribed medicine for the relief of aches and pains as well as a tonic for low spirits and general misery brought about by unremitting physical and economic hardship. The idea of working-class 'stimulant' use was further reinforced in 1834 by the celebrated Public Health reformer, Edwin Chadwick. In evidence before a Select Committee on Drunkenness, he testified to the view that the working classes of the manufacturing towns were given to eating opium in quantity.[20] But Chadwick's evidence contradicted that of the doctors who were called to give evidence to the Factory Inquiry Commission of the same year.[21] In their unanimous testimony they agreed that such practices did not exist in the Factory areas. And in the following decade, it was again reported by a Government Commission of Inquiry that such a practice was not common among the labouring population of the city of Birmingham.[22]

None the less, the mid-century public health campaign's piecemeal enquiries into the extent of opium use, along with its exaggerated and ill-conceived claims about working-class life, Berridge and Edwards maintain, served to sharply define an image of recreational opium use by the working class. Recently Berridge and Edwards have been taken to task by Parssinen[23] over their claim that some form of class-based social control played an important role in shaping nineteenth-century judgements on opium consumption. Opium use emerged as a problem, according to Parssinen, because it became caught up in the legislative aims of public health reformers who, guided by humanitarian considerations, wished to protect the public's health by agitating for improved safety standards in the urban environment. Included among these measures were regulations to control the supply of opium to protect the public against accidental overdoses.

But whatever the motive behind the public health movement's campaign against the open availability of opium and its consumption by the working classes, it did receive support from some quarters of the medical profession during the following decade. In 1840, following his own careful enquiries into the issue, Dr Thompson reported in the *Medical Times* that, 'the consumption of opium is increasing among the working classes to a frightening extent' but the absence of any statistical documentation made it impossible to prove the 'pernicious effects' of opium in a court of law. Working-class consumption as an issue of concern was further compounded by Jonathan Pereira who in 1853 added a new section to the third edition of *Materia Medica* which particularly warned of the dangers arising from the drug's use by the lower classes. By the mid-nineteenth century then, the meaning given to opium consumption and the response it evoked varied with the consumer's class. Working-class consumption was attributed to poor housing conditions and fever epidemics,[24] while its consumption by the middle classes was held to result from their experience of pressure from severe mental distress.[25]

Berridge and Edwards argue the public health movement was further facilitated in its cause by moves to develop the medical and pharmaceutical professions separately. Working-class practices of self-medication stood in diametrical opposition to the rising aims of the middle-class medical and allied professions – to strengthen their control over all forms of medical treatment. It was in their interests to exaggerate the dangers arising from uncontrolled distribution and access to drugs when giving their evidence to the various public health commissions. Whether or not professional interests actually swayed public health reformers is difficult to establish. Undoubtedly the issue of the widespread availability of opium and the relative ease with which one could accidentally or suicidally overdose on the drug was of equally pressing concern to public health reformers. None the less, the collective efforts of both groups had succeeded in raising the profile of opium in the community from that of a legitimate panacea for a range of complaints especially popular among the working classes, to that of a poison whose continued uncontrolled availability was a problem for both the public health reformers concerned by the availability of poisons, and the pharmacists seeking to establish professional control of access to poisons in general, and opium in particular. The first legislative measures designed to regulate opium's availability followed with the passage of the *1868 Poisons and Pharmacy Act* which required opiate-based preparations to be labelled 'poison' and that they be dispensed by a registered pharmacist.

By the latter part of the nineteenth century the public health movement, in league with the medical profession, had succeeded in raising the issue of opium use from one evoking mild curiosity among a scarcely interested public, to one of growing concern. However, towards the end of the century a shift in the response towards the issue of opium consumption had taken place – the point of which was aimed, not at the drug and its availability, but at the opium consumer.

2 The Chinese Opium Wars

THE INDO-CHINESE OPIUM TRADE

The origin of the British-controlled opium trade with China dates back to the early eighteenth century. Opium was first introduced into China by Arab and Turkish traders in the late seventh century. Although the raw opium was occasionally used as an analgesic by the Chinese, the opium poppy *papaver somniferum* was grown in China, until the seventeenth century, as an ornamental plant. When the practice of smoking first reached China opium was mixed with tobacco but the Chinese soon developed their own preferred technique of smoking it on its own in a long, thin-stemmed opium pipe. Following the development of opium smoking as an increasingly popular practice among his people, the Emperor, in 1729, concerned by both the economic consequences of the rapid growth of imported opium and the drug's effects on the nation's health prohibited the sale and smoking of opium.

The opium poppy was also grown in India but was cultivated only for the raw opium it produced. However despite its prohibition the opium trade flourished under the control of the Portuguese who, in the early eighteenth century, found they could import opium from India where the opium poppy was cultivated exclusively for its raw opium, and sell it to China at a considerable profit. To the Portuguese it was considered a legitimate trade in a useful commodity though imports rarely exceeded 200 chests per year.

British attention was drawn to the trade following the conquest of Bengal by Clive (of Clive of India fame) in 1758 when it was discovered that the trade was run exclusively by a ring of wealthy native merchants. But their monopoly was quickly usurped by the East India Company who claimed it for Britain as one of the spoils of war. In 1772, the Governor-General of India, Warren Hastings, took over the monopoly on the company's behalf. He defended this policy with arrogant contempt for the Indian merchants, urging that, 'Opium was not a necessary of life, but a pernicious article of luxury, which ought not be permitted but for the purpose of foreign commerce only, and which the wisdom of the Government should carefully restrain from internal consumption.'[1]

The following year the British East India Company began exporting opium which they grew cheaply and abundantly in the Indian province of Bengal – having already established a depot near Macao where the raw opium could be stored prior to trading it for silver, silks and tea. By 1773 the British had become the leading suppliers to the Chinese market and within twenty years the export of opium had increased five-fold, with a thousand chests of opium per year being imported into China by 1776. But because of its prohibition in China, the East India Company did not carry the opium itself but issued licences to private traders to bring it and other goods from India to China. The traders, in turn, traded the opium with smugglers along the coast, the gold and silver received for the opium was then handed over to the Company against a bill of exchange payable in London in sterling. The gold and silver would then be used by the Company to purchase tea and silks.

By 1781 continually growing demands for opium led Hastings to charter a vessel to extend the trade by selling opium at ports throughout the Far East and particularly those of China. But his initiative upset the East India Company's existing trade arrangements and invoked strong condemnation from its board of directors and in 1786 Hastings faced trial for his actions. The trade however, was too lucrative to be neglected and it continued to be developed by the Company until it was curtailed by the outbreak of hostilities between the Chinese authorities and the British opium merchants, in 1839.

Continuation of the trade despite its earlier prohibition was matched by the issue of further more stringent edicts. In 1796 the Emperor (Kea King) prohibited the importation and sale of opium throughout China. Those caught smoking opium were initially liable to punishment by pillory and lashes with a bamboo cane but he subsequently increased the punishment to imprisonment, transportation and death. Henceforth to the Chinese Government the trade in opium was considered simply as smuggling.

But the trade continued to flourish. In 1800 two thousand chests of opium per year were being imported into China. By 1838 the figure was over thirty-four thousand. The opium was transported in armed vessels and smuggled into the country through bribed customs officials. When this method failed the British merchants resorted to force. By 1836 the situation was becoming intolerable for the Chinese Government which issued an edict which expressly mentioned by name nine of the principal opium merchants in China and insisted on their expulsion from the country. But they stayed put and continued their trade, to the frustration of the Government and the Emperor. Two years later the situation was approaching crisis pitch. A high ranking Chinese official who advised the Emperor to legalise the importation of opium was immediately banished to the country's far province of Tartary. And in a desperate attempt to halt the flow of the drug into China, the Emperor resorted to the most direct of diplomatic channels and wrote to Queen Victoria herself, begging her to forbid the manufacture of opium: 'If you will persist in selling your opium . . . there is not a good or upright man whose head and heart will not burn with indignation at your conduct.'[2] But the letter had no effect. A further proclamation was issued in 1839 which reiterated the earlier demand for the expulsion of the nine principal opium merchants from the country. It further decreed that failure to comply with this demand would result in the opium-carrying ships being forcibly repulsed from the ports. By this stage antagonism between the two sides had increased further with the murder of a Chinese peasant by drunken British sailors. The British Government, distrustful of the Chinese legal system, refused to hand over the guilty men to the courts. The Emperor sent a Commissioner Lin to Canton with authority to deal with the British in the matter of the opium trade. Among his first acts on arrival at the port was to organise the public execution of a Chinese opium smuggler. He then demanded that the opium on board the ships be delivered to his Government for destruction and that the opium traders deliver a promise that opium would not be brought into Canton again. 'I, the Commissioner,' said Lin, 'am sworn to remove utterly this root of misery, nor will I let the foreign vessels have any offshoot left for the root to bud forth again.'[3] When his orders were not complied with he set about blocking the entry to the port and surrounding the opium warehouses thereby trapping inside some two to three hundred British subjects who were involved in the trade.

An ultimatum followed: either the opium traders capitulated to the Chinese Government's demands or all the captured British subjects would be executed. In the event, the Trade Superintendent, Captain Elliot, handed over to the Chinese Commissioner 20 283 chests of opium, valued at over two million pounds sterling. These were subsequently publicly destroyed by mixing the opium with salt and lime. But Lin's victory was only temporary for the trade resumed shortly afterwards and lead inexorably to further conflicts and 'outrages [being] committed on both sides'.

In November 1839 a state of war was declared and 'to our rifles, mortars, and rockets, the Chinese opposed matchlocks, bows and arrows, and shields'. Commenting on the brutality of what he regarded an unjust war, Sir Henry Pottinger, who succeeded Captain Elliot as Superintendent of Trade said, 'It appears that field-pieces loaded with grape had been planted at the end of long narrow streets thronged with men, women, and children, and that they were mowed down like grass, and the gutters flowed with their innocent blood'.[4]

Hostilities continued until August 1842, when the Chinese surrendered to the superior might of the British force and concluded the war by signing the Treaty of Nankin. The Treaty contained a pledge that the British would discourage the smuggling of opium into China and that foreigners would be barred entry into the interior of China. But it also secured a number of concessions for the British. First, that five ports be opened where the British would have residence and trade rights, second, that the Chinese reimburse the British four and a half million pounds sterling to cover the cost of the opium destroyed and for the expense of the war incurred by the merchants, and finally that British nationals in China who were accused of criminal acts had the right to be tried in British courts. It further stipulated that the island of Hong Kong be ceded to the British, who subsequently used it as a strategic base on which to build an opium depot. But despite signing the Treaty, opium continued to be smuggled into mainland China with the full knowledge of the British Government. For their part, British representatives in China repeatedly urged the Chinese Government to legalise the trade, pointing to the vast revenue it would accrue, which would benefit both countries. But the Emperor remained resolute, 'It is true,' he argued, 'I cannot prevent the introduction of the flowing poison; gain-seeking and corrupt men will for profit and sensuality defeat my wishes, but nothing will induce me to derive a revenue from the vice and misery of my people.'[5]

Ill-feeling between the two nations continued and by 1857 they had drifted into a second war particularly more savage than the first. In one scene, *The Times* correspondent reported that within ten minutes 10 000 Chinese had either been captured or killed. And at one stage Canton was laid to siege for twenty-seven hours during which 30 000 people were reported to have been 'burnt out of house and home'. But despite entering Canton as victors the British failed to obtain from the Chinese assurances that the ban on imports of opium would be lifted so the conquering army prepared to lay siege to the capital of China, Pekin. The siege was temporarily averted by the Chinese who, desperate to avoid a repeat of the carnage witnessed in Canton agreed to the signing of the Treaty of Tien-Tsin, on 26 June 1858. The first article of the Treaty cancelled the previous pledge of the 1843 Treaty to discourage the smuggling of opium into China and in a supplement added to the Treaty on 8 November the entry of Indian-grown opium into China was made legal. But the Chinese forcibly resisted the attempts of the British representatives to go to Pekin the following year for the formal ratification of the treaty at the Court of the Emperor and in the renewed hostilities which followed the Treaty was broken. In October 1860, the allied armies had reached the outskirts of Pekin and threatened to bombard it with heavy artillery unless it was surrendered. Against such overwhelming odds the Chinese yielded but not before having secured the Emperor's escape and murdered several British prisoners. As a reprisal for these deaths, the Emperor's Summer Palace was burned down and a large sum of money demanded, in addition to the ratification of the Tien-Tsin Treaty which legalised opium in China. Faced with no feasible alternative the conquered Emperor had little choice and on 24 October it's ratification was publicly proclaimed.

Written into the Treaty of Tien-Tsin was a clause stipulating that every ten years the tariff duty on the imported opium should be subject to review. When the issue did come up for review the Chinese Government took the opportunity to plead their case for the total prohibition of opium once and for all: 'To do away with so great an evil would be a great virtue on England's part,' adding that 'Nothing will be effective but a prohibition to be enforced alike by both parties'.[6] Failing total prohibition they argued for an increase in the duty payable on imported opium, though they believed that the continuation of the trade, which by now had risen to between 50 000 and 60 000 chests a year, despite the increase in revenue it brought, would inexorably 'provoke the judgement of heaven'.

Their petition was ignored until 1876 when the British ambassador in Pekin, Sir Thomas Wade, negotiated a Treaty following a convention in Chefoo, by which Britain agreed to allow China to charge a higher import duty providing no further taxes were levied on it when being distributed throughout the province. It also stipulated that four new ports would be opened to Western trade. Although the Chinese swiftly complied with these requirements, the British Government did not ratify the Treaty until 1885.

3 The Anti-Opium Crusade

Although opium was clearly the issue in the trade wars between China and Britain, at the root of the wars themselves was a conflict of Eastern and Western cultural practices. For centuries the adequate natural resources of China had meant that overseas trade was largely unnecessary, but was tolerated by the ambivalent Chinese as a means of keeping foreigners or 'barbarians' as they called them, under control. Any infringement of restrictions, which they set in order to preserve their culture from foreign and, by implication, detrimental influence would lead to suspension of foreign trade and a boycott of their goods. This action would therefore only harm the 'barbarians'. However, to the British merchants international trade was considered a mutually beneficial practice to all parties concerned and not granted as a favour by one to another. The rules of western trading practice were behind them and were frequently evoked to legitimate their trade in opium which they believed it to be an honest, commercial and exportable commodity. But this attempt to justify their flagrant disregard for Chinese-Sino culture was regarded as immoral not only by the Chinese themselves but by the religiously-inspired founders of a Victorian movement who successfully campaigned for an end to the opium trade with China.

A vociferous member of the movement, Joshua Rowntree captured the objection to the trade with characteristic eloquence. Writing at the turn of the present century, he declared 'The drug, sold as a poison in England, specially prepared to minister to the weakness of the Chinese, has been poured into their country at a rate of a ton per hour for twelve hours of every day for some sixty years.'[1]

THE ANTI-OPIUM MOVEMENT

The history of the anti-opium movement in Britain has been addressed by several commentators: Wu,[2] Owen,[3] Lowes.[4] Notable attempts to analyse these movements, include Brown's[5] brief exposition of the Society for the Suppression of the Opium Trade (SSOT), setting its activities in their imperial context, and

Johnson's[6] interpretation of the opposition to the Indo-Chinese trade which he details as a conflict between the different moral persuasions of the anti- and pro-opium lobbies. The anti-opium organisations were profoundly disturbed by political and economic expediencies which were evoked by the opium merchants to legitimate their trade. The anti-opium campaigners' objections lay in their belief that opium, when consumed for non-medical purposes, i.e. gratuitously and not for any specific ailment, was evil, and that the Chinese Government, recognising this, had a right to block its importation on moral grounds. When it continued to be forced upon them despite Chinese protestations British anti-opiumists embarked on numerous campaigns with a characteristic zealous self-righteousness, in order to make good what they perceived as an immoral trading practice, guided in their endeavours by their rationale that nothing could be politically right when morally wrong. The first sporadic protests against the trade date back to the first Opium War (1839–43). In 1840, an 'Anti-Opium Society' was responsible for the publication of W. S. Fry's *Facts and Evidence Relating to the Opium Trade with China*. Its rationale for agitation was eloquently summarised by Gladstone – Prime Minister of the day – who, denouncing a war into which the government had blundered, wrote:

> They [The Chinese] gave you [The British Merchants in Opium] to abandon your contraband trade [*sic*]. When they found that you would not, they had a right to drive you from their coasts, in account of your obstinacy in persisting in this infamous and atrocious traffic. You allow your Agent to aid and abet those who were concerned in carrying on that trade. A war more unjust in its origins, a war more calculated to cover this country with permanent disgrace, I do not know, and have not read of.[7]

Three years later Lord Shaftsbury, who also strongly opposed the trade, was urged by two Quakers to introduce a resolution to Parliament which called for the termination of the trade. This he did, but subsequently withdrew. However in 1855 as chairman of a 'Committee formed to sever all connections of the English people and its government with the opium trade' he re-introduced it, but it was defeated. In 1857 Shaftsbury went on to seek the House of Lords' judgement on the legality of the East India Company's monopolistic trade in opium and further asked if this did not go against the 1842 Treaty. Their conclusions, although ruling against Shaftsbury, however did accept that the spirit of the Treaty was being violated. Curiously, Shaftsbury's committee failed to capitalise on this admission and, shortly after, it disappeared, possibly because of inadequate funding or a lack of interest.

The issue was brought to the attention of the Quakers again in 1858. During one of their business meetings, the issue was recorded as having 'Engaged the deep feelings of the meeting'; and agitative action against the trade, in the form of a memorial to the Government, was pledged.[8] Two reformist societies subsequently formed by the Quakers; the Aborigines Protection Society and the Society for the Suppression of Opium Smuggling were particularly instrumental in leading attitudes on the trade during the mid-Victorian era though, like so many other movements of the era, they disappeared into obscurity shortly after they emerged. In all during the nineteenth century there existed at least three specifically anti-opium societies each with a life of twenty-five years or more.[9]

THE SOCIETY FOR THE SUPPRESSION OF THE OPIUM TRADE

Most prominent among these was the Anglo-Oriental Society for the Suppression of the Opium Trade (SSOT – the 'Anglo-Oriental' was soon dropped from the title). The Society was significantly different from the others, not least because it was the first well led and financed of its kind, giving an organisational focus to the hitherto sporadic protests by the anti-opium movement as a whole. Moreover, for almost fifty years its members – who were characteristically strong moral enforcers committed to using political practices to change what they perceived as wrong – had waged an unremitting and ultimately successful campaign against the British Government's foreign opium trade policy.

The Society was founded on 14 November 1874, by Edward Pease, a wealthy northern industrialist and Quaker who also founded the Stockton to Darlington Railway and the Peace Society. Its impetus derived from a public meeting held in the same year in Birmingham, which was organised by a local Quaker, Thomas Reynolds. Reynolds, along with other moral reformists, regarded the exploitative practices endorsed by British colonial policies as distasteful, and particularly abhorred the use of force to export opium to China. The meeting was intended to draw the public's attention to a trade which had previously aroused little concern. But it was Edward Pease, offering prizes up to two hundred pounds for the best essay on the subject of 'British opium policy and its results to India and China', who most seriously disturbed the 'almost total silence and oblivion into which this dark subject had been too easily allowed to sink'.[10]

The Quaker-dominated meeting resolved to form an anti-opium committee and from it in November, the London-based SSOT was formed. The Society gathered momentum in early 1875 with receipt of its initial funding, the bulk of which came from Quakers and especially the Pease family. Edward Pease founded the Society with an initial donation of one thousand pounds, and provided an annual subscription of two hundred pounds until his death in 1880. Edward's brother, Arthur, provided one hundred pounds annually. Two other Quakers also pledged sizable annual subscriptions of two hundred and fifty pounds: Thomas Hansbury, a pharmaceutical merchant who held investments in China, and Arthur Albright, a Birmingham merchant. But it was Edward's grandson, Joseph Whitwell Pease, who went on to underwrite the Society's efforts for nearly thirty years, until his death in 1903.

The Society's forty-six man General Council, presided over by the Earl of Shaftsbury, included seventeen members of Parliament, eighteen ecclesiastical ministers and several other distinguished members: Thomas Barnardo, the London philanthropist and founder of Dr Barnardo Homes; Edward Bains, the educational reformer; and Thomas Hughes, Liberal MP and author of *Tom Brown's Schooldays*. The only non-Quaker to perform an influential role in the SSOT was F. Storrs-Turner, an experienced missionary in China, who was appointed the Society's first secretary.

Storrs-Turner was also made editor of the Society's journal *Friend of China*, which provided a significant forum for the anti-opium movement as a whole. Under its masthead which carried the epigraph 'Righteousness exalteth a nation, but sin is a reproach to any people' was published the decisions of the Society's executive committee, the proceedings from the Society's annual meetings and details of forthcoming public meetings up and down the country, held under the auspices of the SSOT.[11] The

SOCIETY FOR THE SUPPRESSION OF THE OPIUM TRADE.

THE

ANNUAL MEETING

WILL BE HELD AT

EXETER HALL,

On TUESDAY, May 31st, 1892, at 7 p.m.,

THE PRESIDENT,

SIR JOSEPH W. PEASE, BART, M.P.

Will occupy the Chair, and Addresses will be delivered by

Mr. CHEOK HONG CHEONG, of Melbourne,

(Superintendent of Church Missions to the Chinese in Victoria), who is about to return to Australia,

Rev. CANON WILBERFORCE, M.A., Rev. PROFESSOR LEGGE, D.D. (of Oxford),

LADY HENRY SOMERSET,

(President of the British Women's Temperance Association),

Miss LUCY E. GUINNESS, (of the Women's Anti-Opium Urgency League),

Dr. DONALD MORISON, (of Rampore Bauleah, Bengal),

AND

Rev. JOSEPH S. ADAMS,

(17 years Missionary in Upper Burma and Inland China).

ADMISSION FREE.

A FEW SEATS WILL BE RESERVED, PRICE 1s.

Tickets for which may be obtained at Exeter Hall, from Messrs. Dyer Brothers, 31, Paternoster Square, E.C.; Miss Braithwaite, Hon. Sec. Women's Anti-Opium Urgency League, 312, Camden Road, N.; or Mr. J. G. Alexander, Secretary of the Society, Broadway Chambers, Westminster, S.W.

ON THE SAME DAY,

A PRAYER MEETING

WILL BE HELD AT THE

Friends' Meeting House, St. Martin's Lane, near Charing Cross

Commencing at 11 a.m. SUBJECTS:

11 to 12—"The Opium Trade a Hindrance to Missionary Effort."

Chairman:—BENJAMIN BROOMHALL, Esq.

(Secretary of the China Inland Mission).

12 to 1—"The Opium Trade a National Reproach."

Chairman:—Rev. F. B. MEYER, B.A.

A Conference on the Medical Aspects of the Opium Question,

WILL BE HELD AT THE

FRIENDS' MEETING HOUSE, at 3 p.m., when Papers will be read by

JAMES L. MAXWELL, Esq., M.D.

(Secretary of the Medical Missionary Association, formerly Medical Missionary in Formosa); and

DONALD MORISON, Esq., M.D. (*of Rampore Bauleah, Bengal*).

Full opportunity for discussion will be afforded at this Conference.

names of those who had donated financial support with details of the amount were occasionally included together with correspondence from other anti-opium organisations from as far afield as Australia, New Zealand and Japan. It also regularly published resolutions tabled in the House of Commons by its members, though most notably by the Society's one-time president, Sir Joseph Whitwell Pease.

Apart from informing and co-ordinating the efforts of the Society's members, the journal also served as a mouthpiece for the opinions of the influential and attracted articles and comments from contributors representing a broad spectrum of interests in the growing debate on opium. Speeches and letters from missionaries in China, from MPs, from Archbishops, from Lord Mayors and from eminent figures in the medical profession, testifying to the harmful consequences of the trade for both the Chinese and the British were reproduced alongside features culled from popular newspapers and magazines, some of which were distinctly pro-opium. *The Times* of 11 November 1892 for instance, argued that the anti-opiumists were 'Supersensitive Christians', 'ludicrous' and 'Pharisees of an extremely odious kind' The editor continued that 'China used opium for a thousand years before the English set foot in India, and she is not debauched yet.'

In March 1875 the *Friend of China*, circulated monthly and eventually running to thirty-two volumes, was first published. In it the Society, maintaining that Chinese dependence on opium had retarded the advances of legitimate trade, published its major lines of attack against the trade. It claimed that (a) Britain forced opium on China, (b) Revenue was the sole reason for continuing the trade, (c) Prohibition except for medical purposes was the Society's long-range goal, (d) Everyone (except the British Government's India Office) agreed that opium is evil, (e) Opium could not be consumed in moderation, and (f) Opium physically and morally destroyed the user. Articles from scientific journals and periodically-reported government policy decisions together with statistics depicting increases in exports of opium and a rise in its consumption in China were also regularly reprinted in *Friend of China*.

Following through these lines of attack with several years of anti-drug sermons, tracts and further resolutions the SSOT's campaign began to produce results. A resolution by Sir Joseph Whitwell Pease asking the British Government to treat China as an 'independent state, having the right to arrange its own import duties' although originally defeated in Parliament by a majority of sixty votes was subesquently renegotiated in 1885. From these negotiations it was decided that the Chinese would henceforth be regarded by the British government as equals who were free to demand higher import duties on opium. The decision however owed more to the expediencies of politics, than to the SSOT's moral crusade.[12]

None the less, the SSOT in conjunction with its affiliated organisations, the Christian Union for the Severance of the Connection of the British Empire, Friends' Anti-Opium Committee for Suffering, Anti-opium Urgency Committee and the Women's Anti-opium Urgency Committee, by the early twentieth century had, between them, worn down the defenders of the opium trade through attrition. Its success as a moral pressure group was evident in May 1906 by the unanimously approved passage through the House of Commons of a resolution calling for a speedy close of the Indo-Chinese opium trade; whereas similar motions by Joseph Whitwell Pease, in 1875 and 1883 had previously failed by a two to one majority. The Society's extensive political activities were clearly instrumental in achieving its aims. But the development of an international response towards narcotics control intitiated at a series of international meetings beginning in Shanghai in 1909, was also partly responsible for ensuring its success. However, the significance of international narcotics control for domestic drugs policy should not be overstated.[13]

Britain was in fact an unwilling participant in the first of these meetings and attended largely because of American pressure to do so. Diplomatic manoeuvrings culminating in 1907 with the British Government's promise of a gradual termination of the opium trade with China by 1917 meant that as regards Great Britain there was no evident need for further action by the SSOT. Its task near completed, the SSOT eventually disbanded in 1917. In the 42nd and final report of the Society, presented at a meeting held in Caxton Hall on 19 April, Joseph Alexander, the Society's honorary secretary, referred to certain areas where the sale of opium for non-medical purposes continued: a practice which he maintained, called for the Society's continued efforts. Therefore at the closure of the SSOT a Vigilance Committee was established which aimed (1) to continue the work of the SSOT, (2) to complete the campaign against the opium trade where it persisted, (3) to collect information in regard to misuse of opium and related drugs; and to exercise particular diligence against the recurrence of the trade in areas where it appears suppressed, and (4) to intervene actively wherever such action appears necessary. But with the SSOT's major battle well behind them the issue of the opium trade had already slipped from the public's eye and the Committee sank quickly into obscurity.

4 Constructing Addiction as a Moral Failing

DESCRIBING ADDICTION AS A 'MORAL FAILING'

The aim of the SSOT, to convince the British public of the harm inflicted on the Chinese by the continuance of the opium trade, was reiterated in each issue of the *Friend of China*. They were aided considerably in their propagandist efforts by reports which filtered back from medical missionaries in China who testified to the injurious effects of opium on the indigenous population. From their daily contact with the opium-using Chinese they perceived the harm to result from the favoured Chinese recreational practice of ingesting opium through smoking; something practically unheard of in Britain. Reprinted wholesale in the *Friend of China*, (and frequently adjacent to pro-opium testimonies) these missionaries documented their observations of the effects of opium smoking under several headings, including social and physical as well as spiritual. The Rev. Griffiths John, a medical missionary with several years' experience of working in China, concluded that the physical effects on the Chinese following 'immoderate' consumption for opium smoking,

> undermines the Constitution, ruins the health, and shortens the life of the smoker . . . The appetite becomes more intense and insatiable every day; the smallest use leads infallibly to an intemperate use; gradually it so weakens the system that it becomes an easy prey to diseases of all kinds. As soon as the means of gratification are exhausted, or the supply of the necessaries of life is diminished, death appears. A strenuous attempt to break off the habit induces an incurable opium diarrhoea, which often proves fatal . . . In the case of those who are in mid way circumstances, and who have got inured to the habit, the enervating effects are such that they become after a time unable to attend to their ordinary advocations. They then lose their situations, or their business fails, and they are reduced to necessity. Gradually they part with their little property, furni-

> ture, clothes, until they come to the level of the labouring poor, without those energetic habits which might otherwise form the ground of support. Among the lower classes, those who indulge in the use of opium are reduced to abject poverty sooner than the preceeding. Having nothing to dispose of in the shape of property, furniture or clothes, their wives and children are sold to supply their ever-increasing appetite for the drug, and when these are gone, with greatly diminished strength for labour, they can no longer earn sufficient for their own wants, and are obliged to beg for their daily bread.[1]

Similar accounts can be drawn from almost any issue of the *Friend of China*, and not just from medical missionaries. Sir Rutherford Alcock, British Foreign Minister in China during the 1860s, in a summary of the effects of opium smoking on the Chinese before a Parliamentary Commission on Opium, reported opium users who were turned into 'moral criminals'. 'This' he argued, 'is the conclusion to which a calm and impartial survey of all accessible testimony on the subject has led the great majority of Englishmen who have considered the question.'[2]

Alcock and his fellow commentators however, only emphasised the deleterious effects from the peculiarly foreign practice of *smoking* opium while ingesting opium through the stomach was considered a therapeutic practice and therefore acceptable. In 1888 Canon Worburton reported in *Friend of China* on enquiries of the day which purported to show that opium consumed by peasants in the fen district of Eastern England was taken on medical advice as a preventive measure against such common complaints as pleurisy and so forth.[3] Opium smoking on the other hand was altogether a different matter. Witnesses presented before the Committee on the Opium Question repeatedly described accounts of the emaciated opium smoker who went, 'off into a sort of absolute unconsciousness after two whiffs' and who only returned to consciousness when the effects of the 'whiffs' wore off.[4]

This image of the opium-dependent Chinese peasant was constantly evoked in *Friend of China* to reinforce the drug's 'pernicious effects': 'There is nothing too mean or corrupt for him to attempt. He will lie, cheat, and steal, without the faintest sense of shame or wrong. He may not knock about his wife and children, as the dram-drinker does, for opium does not work in that direction exactly, but he will in cold blood sell his wife, starve his children, and steal the clothes of the backs of his aged parents, and cause them to die from cold.'[5]

To graphically reinforce the dangers associated with opium smoking, the SSOT published, as an occasional supplement to their journal, pamphlets of colour illustrations depicting the opium smoker's career which carried such provocative titles as, 'From the ruddy youth inhaling his first pipe, to living skeleton clothed in rags'.[6]

The physical effects apart however, 'the crowning evil of all', according to the Rev.J.C. Kerr MD was the 'deterioration of the moral faculty'. Eyewitness testimonies of opium smokers who have consequently lost their 'regard for truth', for 'right' and thus for 'nobility', who had 'blunted moral natures' and in whom 'natural affection' had died, thus abounded throughout each issue of *Friend of China*. Although these testimonies came from informed religious, medical and diplomatic sources, underpinning them all was the religiously-inspired notion of opium smoking as an immoral vice. Each opium-smoking Chinese peasant was therefore individually responsible for his own moral debasement.

FROM VICE TO MORAL PATHOLOGY

As the SSOT's campaign gathered momentum, its initial concern with the Chinese practice of smoking opium was gradually extended to all modes of opium use. By the end of the nineteenth century, the Society's campaign against British involvement in the opium trade had succeeded in raising the issue of the non-medical use of opium to the level of a national concern. But its success did not lie simply in convincing the British public that opium's addictive properties required it to be subject to some form of legislative control; the Medical and Pharmaceutical professions had already established this as a basis for the 1868 Pharmacy Act. The SSOT's achievement in raising public concern over opium use rested instead on the ability of its founder members to use a technical language to examine the *cause* of opium dependence, instead of an everyday language which could just *describe* its observed effects. Using their technical language the founders of the SSOT attributed to opium a particular property the kind of which had not been previously considered; the property of impairing the habitual user, not just physically, but also morally. In other words this technical language described the manifest symptoms of opium dependence as those of a 'vice' but analysed its aetiology in terms of a pathologically impaired moral faculty.

However odd their reasoning may have appeared to others, to the founders of the SSOT this made sound sense. It could do so because they subscribed to Quaker doctrine which was founded on the principle that an individual's 'soul' should be regarded to all intent and purpose as a physical entity like, for example, a person's body. In other words, they could speak of a 'material soul'. Unlike conventional religious sects where the moral faculty exists on a spiritual plane, the Quakers considered it to exist on a physical plane. For Quakers the path to righteousness was therefore marked not by prayer, as with many nineteenth-century conformist religious sects, but by the pursuit of those activities nourishing the soul's moral faculty, such as simplicity, industriousness, moderation, and active recognition of one's material and spiritual responsibilities. The Quaker founders of the SSOT therefore spoke of opium, when taken as a 'sensual indulgence' or 'stimulant' (which undermined the pursuit of these activities) as extremely injurious to the 'soul'. Those who became dependent on it were deemed to have suffered a breakdown of the 'normal' self-restraining function of an individual which resulted in the irresponsible denial of one's own morality.

The Society's campaign, by the turn of the century, had popularised the view that the opium-dependent individual – whether a Chinese peasant addicted to the opium pipe or a Laudanum-dependent British labourer – by virtue of the actions of the opium on the soul was thus morally debased. Using this language it became possible for the members of the SSOT to describe those dependent on opium as wilfully adopting a course of self-destruction while fully aware of its probable consequences: in other words, 'willing victims'.

The notion of debilitated 'willing victims' whose dependence on opium resulted in their 'enfeebled will', 'shattered constitution', 'deteriorated moral character', 'lost moral obligation' 'moral obliquity' and 'blunted moral sense' provided the theme of the SSOT's campaign which resonated throughout the crusade. In his address to the annual meeting of the SSOT in 1886, the chairman, encapsulating this theme, denounced the seductive properties of opium on the moral faculty, 'at first producing a higher intellectual activity, a greater mental brightness and cleverness than the individual possibly ever enjoyed before: giving him vivacity of speech, even more brilliancy in the expression of his countenance and a greater eloquence to his tongue. After a time, however, it begins to sap his moral nature, and leads him steadily and steadily downwards in the path of demoralisation'. Echoing this sentiment, Joseph Whitwell Pease, the Society's one time President, was moved to write of opium dependence, 'By it human life is shorn of every vestige of nobility and moral responsibility. The mind is rendered insentiate to every enobling desire or sentiment, and the moral nature of man is unfathomably degraded to an even greater depth of brutishness.'[7] Alfred Dyer, a fellow Quaker and Society member, maintained the habit 'pre-eminently destroys the power of the will'.[8]

First-hand experience of opiates' demoralising effects taken from popular magazines of the day were frequently republished as the SSOT's pamphlets. The case of an addicted doctor's fight against these effects, reprinted in *Friend of China* and separately as a leaflet points up the effects of opiates on the moral faculty of even the most respectable of citizens.

> Sir, – when working for my graduate's degree in medicine, in Aberdeen in 1868, I contracted the habit of taking opium. I begun by small doses of laudanum as a remedy for tic – dental in its origin and which was quite cured by the dentist in due course. I continued the laudanum because it made my brain clear, kept me warm in the cold weather of that winter, and because I liked it. I began it on my birthday, January 3rd, and by the middle of April I was taking thirteen grains of opium a day. I said quite airily to a friend who lived with me that I should break it off on one night, and should select the night I travelled home to London. I believed I could do so: I little knew the hold the drug had on me. By the time we reached Perth I was very nearly raving mad. I broke my journey there, and managed, by some sort of falsification of facts, to get enough laudanum to carry me on to Edinburgh. There I told fresh lies, and replenished my stock of laudanum. Again, at York, I got some more, and arrived in London I went in for a perfect opium debauch [*sic*]. I went home, and for a month I was happy, but had sadly increased my dosage, – happily, till one day I realised

> that my word was no longer a symbol of truth, and the moral nature I had not quite drowned leapt up in the dark and called me 'liar!' to my face. Then I awoke, and for the first time for many a day I prayed. Then also came the resolve, the determined resolve, come what may, to be done with this damnable tyranny.

Therefore, only by virtue of having partly retained his moral faculty in fact was the doctor able to successfully withdraw from the drug, and then, not without some trauma. 'The craving seemed to me a palpable shape that walked beside me – a presence that outran me and lost me, and came back to me like a faithful dog, that would not lose or leave me, that I could not leave or lose! Sometimes I sang, sometimes I raved and swore, sometimes I prayed and wept, but never once, thank God, did my resolution falter . . . Since that day I have never touched it, and have never been tempted to touch it.'[9]

By the end of the century it was not just the society's founding members who described the aetiology in terms of a pathologically debilitated will. Eye witness accounts of opium dependence in China which had previously described a 'vice' had also adopted the language of the SSOT's founders. The Rev. Johns for example, argued that opium paralysed the moral nature and prostrated the will, bedimmed the moral vision and blunted the moral sentiment.[10] Theodore Cooke Taylor MP argued in the same vein that opium actually made people unmoral, maintaining that it 'weakens every fibre of their moral being and leaves them physical and moral wrecks'.[11] And in evidence before the Royal Commission on Opium in 1895 Dr Mookerjee stated that opium, 'most certainly tarnishes the moral nature of man, weakening his mental control over his will, and thus causing him to be the prey of the evil and vicious habits of lying and stealing.' Dr Manohar Prasdad Tewarie concurred with this view when also called to give evidence, adding that 'Its use in any of its forms deadens the intellect.'[12]

PATHOLOGISING THE SOUL

Since opium use was first documented the drug's pharmacological properties have been described in terms of their psychological and physical effects on the mind and body. Earlier in the nineteenth century, speculative reasoning had led some moralists to associate the non-medical use of opium with an immoral state of vice, but as I have suggested, it was the SSOT's founder members who ventured to *analyse* this particular mode of use in terms of an impaired moral faculty. They argued that apart from the observable effects of opium on the individual such as alterations in physiological functioning and mood, when opiates were taken for non-medical purposes, they deleteriorily affected that which could not be directly observed: the individual's moral faculty. The metaphor of a 'material soul' was clearly central to the existence of what might be loosely termed this 'moral pathological' model of addiction in that it allowed the SSOT's founders to implicate the pharmacological effects of opium on the celestial body of the soul with their claim that opiates fostered a state of immorality by undermining self-restraint. But how was it possible for others who did not belong to the SSOT to take seriously the claim that the cause of non-medical use of opium was to be located in some pathologically impaired 'moral faculty'?

It is not the claim as such which is significant here, but the founders of the SSOT who made it and could expect the public to take their claim seriously, an ability which may be attributed to the hallmark of their organisation: their standing as Quakers. This above all else distinguished their organisation from similar ones within the anti-opium movement.

5 Opium and the Quakers

QUAKERS: A PECULIAR PEOPLE

With the single exception of Storrs-Turner, the founders of the Society were also members of the Quakers' organising body, the Society of Friends. Membership to this august body ensured an elevated status in the community but was strictly controlled and conferred only on those who had satisfactorily met the criteria of competence for, and knowledge of, the Quakers' mission of divinely appointed guardians of moral standards. Members were therefore expected to regularly attend Quaker meetings;[1] and their social conduct and spiritual inspiration was compatible with other Quakers. Except for those who could claim birthright membership, i.e. born of two Quaker parents in good standing with these meetings, prospective candidates to the sect had to endure a complex and arduous 'right of passage'. Having made an initial application for membership, applicants would be visited in their homes by two long established 'Friends', elders of the sect, who would conduct a scrutinising interview to ascertain elegibility. Should this prove satisfactory the prospective members would be invited to attend one of the monthly meetings where these applicants would be asked to 'give of their experience'. This involved testifying to their recognition of a 'divine calling', a religious inspiration which moved them to seek conversion. Divine knowledge and competence however were invariably synonymous. J. Whitwell Pease himself testified to this in an impassioned plea for the termination of the opium trade at a public meeting of the SSOT. 'Surely', he argued, 'as a Christian country, in the light of that religion which we believe comes down from Heaven not merely to illuminate the hearts of men, but to act upon the sense of duty in every man, we ought to be able to accomplish a revolution in a revenue which most of us, having looked into the question, say could be very well dispensed with.'[2]

Knowledge of this 'divine calling' was a central principle of Quakerism. On the basis of it the Quaker founders of the SSOT, as highly esteemed guardians of public morality, could question the spiritual health of the community in a way no other nineteenth-century moralists could. Moreover, they received their authority to do so from the community they served. Using their divinely inspired wisdom it was possible for Quakers to 'see' beneath the level of appearances to the moral faculty, and to know whether or not certain physical actions affected it. On the basis of this divine calling, or as it was known in Quaker circles, 'inner light', devout Quakers believed themselves to possess a wisdom that enabled them to see beyond the appearance of things to their essence. This belief was sharpened in issues of commercial business in which many nineteenth-century Quakers were involved. Their own business transactions exemplified propriety and took issue with those which, like the opium trade, they believed did not. Although the trade appeared a legitimate commercial enterprise the Quaker founders of the SSOT detected that beneath this veneer of respectability the trade had a debilitating effect on morality. Even gaming places, horse races and playhouses were subject to the close scrutiny of Friends who saw them as containing an intrinsic evil and referred to them as, 'those nurseries of debauchery and wickedness'.[3]

This 'wisdom' played a central part in formulating opium's effects in terms of a pathologised moral faculty. The earliest spokesman for this concept was the founder of the SSOT Edward Pease. The Darlington Monthly Meeting in its tribute to Pease on his death in 1880 acknowledging his privileged insight, recorded:

> His communications were accompanied by great power and feeling; they were marked by earnestness, simplicity and happy illustrations, and were very instructive as showing the great use and benefit of employing Scripture, one part throwing light upon the other. He was concerned faithfully to preach the council of God, and at all times to speak under the immediate guidance of the Holy Spirit.[4]

This notion of Quakers as a sect apart continued well into the nineteenth century. Quakers, or 'Friends' as they were known to their fellow Quakers, believed themselves to be a 'peculiar people' whose traditions derived from the experience and writings of their seventeenth-century founders, including George Fox (1624–1691). During the nineteenth century they could be distinguished by their style of dress, the man by his collarless coat and broad-brimmed hat, the woman by her 'Quaker' bonnet and choice of plain unornamented clothes in dark colours;[5] their speech, referring to (Sun)day as 'first day', (Mon)day as 'second day' and so on in order to avoid all references to paganism; and their rules of etiquette which included forbidding the man's removal of his hat even when dictated to do so by custom. And until the late nineteenth century, marriage to non-Quakers ('marriage out' in Quaker terminology) was strictly prohibited on pain of expulsion.

Assertive action directed against certain conformist practices further compounded the Quaker's identity as that of a separatist status group. For example, Quakers had disapproved of the established Church from the movement's earliest days and refused to pay parish taxes levied to cover the Church's expenses, adopting a policy of passive resistance whereby they permitted part of their goods, to the cost of these unpaid taxes, to be confiscated in lieu. They assumed a similar separatist stance over the issue of warfare to which they were also opposed. The Boer war, and most importantly conscription during the First World War, did expose a lack of unanimity on the issue and drove some members from its ranks, but until the late nineteenth century their non-conformity projected the Quakers' image as a sect of distinct principles.

Paramount among these was their commitment to putting down evil wherever it was detected, a point clearly made in an 1878 issue of the Quakers' monthly journal, *The Friend*, 'The palpable evils afflicting humanity in any part of the earth are the topics that most closely occupy the thoughts of Friends everywhere'. Such a proud boast might possibly not have been made with equal justification by any other denomination. In their crusades for moral reform the front line of attack against evil involved the first principle of Quakerism; 'Great is the Force of Example'.[6]

Their own style of life provided at all times a clear, albeit extremely puritan, example of virtuosity, frugality and piety. But Quakers were also well aware that some evils occasionally necessitated a more positive, direct action; and their nineteenth-century organisation was not without teeth. Indeed they ceaselessly agitated for many just causes in the form of powerful and remarkably successful pressure groups; and were widely recognised as effective allies, bringing pressure to bear from three modes of political action. Petitioning was especially popular among Victorian Friends as a principal source of extra-Parliamentary influence. But on matters which Quakers considered particularly important, they campaigned on two additional fronts: direct pressure exerted on constituency MPs, and deputations sent to parliamentary ministers. Both strategies were used to considerable effect in the SSOT's campaign, which was undoubtedly aided by the election in 1865 of Joseph Whitwell Pease, the Society's one time President, as a Liberal member of Parliament for South Durham until 1885 and then for Barnard Castle.

The status of the SSOT's members also owed much to its wealthier members' philanthropy. Quaker members were directed to the doctrine of avoidance of luxuries, of exhibiting pride, of undue expenditure, of self-indulgence and were instead encouraged in the adoption of the principle of moderation in all things. The doctrine also staunchly advocated as particularly virtuous, free trading practices and economic gain, so long as no moral harm was incurred. During the nineteenth century, such practices could and indeed did lead to the accumulation of great amounts of wealth, not least by the Quakers, who were deemed as 'a shrewd race in matters of money and business'.[7] The vast riches of the Pease Family, for example, derived from their cotton manufacturing business in the North of England.[8] The two seemingly incompatible practices of piety and accumulated wealth were readily reconciled by prosperous Quakers who, in order to remain in accord with the dictates of their doctrine and so maintain their standing both in their own community and the social community beyond, became magnificently benevolent philanthropists. So wealthy Quakers of great business ability, who had devoted their earlier years to the accumulation of wealth, devoted their latter years to dispersing it (often under great secrecy in order to avoid a show of grandiosity and maintain the Quakers' chastened image), under the pious aspiration that, 'The best recreation of a Christian is the relief of distress'.[9] Indeed by the mid-nineteenth century, philanthropy had become almost an hereditary duty among many wealthy Quaker families (The Pease family's financial commitment to the SSOT being a notable example).

The Quaker doctrine of frugality, the munificent philanthropic acts by the Society's wealthier members, and the Quaker self-prescribed role of the poor's prime benefactor all contributed to their moral reformist status. Even those who took exception to Quakers' wealth acknowledged the virtuous uses to which it was often put. An anonymous author who equated the Friends' characteristic wealth with the 'surest sign of their decadence' was given to admit that, 'Their charity is large, universal, and as wide as suffering humanity; it asks no questions about creed, or age, or sex, or colour'.[10]

Their wealth apart, Quakers were admired as a prestigious and immensely respectable religious sect. Their eccentric customs did on occasion provoke the non-Quaker, but 'Friends' were usually regarded as people of 'public spirit, upright, sincere, claiming men's respect if they cannot share their convictions'.[11] Joseph Pease (1799–1872), (father of Joseph Whitwell Pease) the first Quaker to sit in Parliament was observed to be 'a frequent speaker on matters of social and political reform, always avoiding the use of titles when addressing the house, and retaining his Quaker dress'.[12]

Even the Quakers' reputation for quaintness, passive suffering and the 'appearance of the women like goddesses of innocence and purity' were a source of respect and a mark of their status. Such public affirmation of the Quaker's role as a staunch, committed moral guardian served to compound further their elevated status in the community.

Quakerism during the nineteenth century then became synonymous with respectability which probably owed much to their success in business. Indeed Quakers were regarded as meaning business in every sense of the word. In matters of public morality, just as with their business dealings they were not given to idle speculation. When they spoke out on any issue they measured their words with meticulous care believing their knowledge to be divinely inspired. The same meticulous care was observed by Edward Pease and his fellow founders of the SSOT when making their claim that addiction was caused by a pathologically debilitated will. They were serious in their claim and as Quakers their claim was also taken seriously. But how was it that addiction had not been formulated in this way earlier, when opium had been used extensively throughout Great Britain since the early nineteenth century? To formulate the cause of addiction in these terms requires the effects of opium to be observed repeatedly, and for these observations to be recorded systematically in order that an overall picture of these effects may be built up. Such techniques for this form of surveillance were built into the organisational structure of the Quaker Society of Friends and were incorporated into the SSOT thus enabling Pease and his associates to 'see' beneath the surface effects of compulsive opium use to its underlaying cause.

THE SOCIETY OF FRIENDS' ORGANISATIONAL STRUCTURE

The organisational structure of the Society of Friends was a highly regarded feature of nineteenth-century Quakerism. 'Their internal government was much admired, their poor are supported without parochial aid, and their industry and sobriety are deserving of imitation.'[13] Indeed the backbone of the Society of Friends comprised a hierarchical arrangement of 'business meetings'. At the bottom were the weekly Preparative Meetings, each comprised of one or several local congregations, whose tasks included collating information on births and deaths in the local Quaker population. But in the main they were primarily concerned with preparing business matters for the Monthly Meetings. These covered a larger area and were attended by Quakers from one or more counties. In organisational terms they were significantly more important than weekly meetings, exercising a number of executive functions such as processing applications for membership and dealing with reported incidences of Quaker delinquency. Quarterly Meetings had comparatively few functions and their *raison d'etre* was mainly to act as a channel of communication between Monthly and Yearly Meetings and to elect a representative to attend the latter. The Yearly Meeting, situated at the top of the Quaker's organisational pyramid, was held in London, and its activities may be likened to the National Assembly of the British Quaker movement.

The organisational arrangement of these business meetings provided an effective channel of communication between the various Quaker congregations and conveyed information about the state and condition of Quakerism throughout the whole country. It also served to unify the Society's membership and widen its base. But decisions to revise Quaker doctrine, and to establish their position on social and political issues were ordinarily made on a yearly basis, and there was an evident need for a standing committee to deal with more immediate issues as they arose throughout the year.

This function was assumed by the Meeting for Sufferings. Unlike other meetings, these were not open to the whole membership, but attendance was limited by office and consisted of elders and ministers, though they occasionally included representatives from the Quarterly Meetings. Meetings for Sufferings (a curious title considering their function) were invariably well attended but were too large to perform effectively and so delegated much of their work to various sub-committees. Subsequent to their formal recognition in 1833 as executive committees of the Yearly Meeting, these Meetings played a vastly important role in the Society of Friends' nineteenth-century functioning. Their tasks included raising and administering special funds when so instructed by the Yearly Meeting; but their primary function was surveillance. As Isichei notes in her detailed description of nineteenth-century Quakers, 'It kept an eagle eye on parliamentary proceedings and intervened instantly when an issue came up which bore on Quaker interests. [it] . . . watched over English ministers abroad [and] on a multitude of occasions it spoke and acted for Quakerism as no other body could.'[14]

The Meeting for Sufferings reported observations by Quakers up and down the country of instances of immoral behaviour; their nature and form, the type of person engaging in such activities, their class, ethnic origin and such, and observations of correlative activities such as crime. These filtered up the Society's organisational structure and depicted to the Yearly Meeting the geographical and social distribution of vices, and the frequency with which they emerged as issues of concern. Using these techniques of surveillance it was possible for Quakers to observe and record instances of immorality which recurred time and again. This enabled them to construct a national picture of the nature, extent of and, more importantly, to establish a cause associated with, such outbreaks of immoral practices.

Objections to the Indo-Chinese Opium Trade were reported to the Yearly Meetings and committed the Society of Friends to direct action in rousing anti-opium sentiment. A three-pronged campaign was launched by the Society detailing the immorality of continuing the trade, the demoralising effects on the Chinese, and the attendant effects of the trade on the morals of the British nation.[15] It was in a Meeting for Sufferings in 1858 that the Quakers' attention to the Opium Trade was first drawn, having 'engaged the deep feelings of this meeting'.[16] The issue was again raised by the Meeting for Sufferings in 1877, which pledged support for the Emperor of China's anti-opium stance. Three years later, at a monthly meeting of the Society of Friends held in London, the question of the duty of the Society with regard to the Opium traffic was considered again. The discussion, opened by

Sir Edward Fry, a leading opponent of the trade and an active member of the SSOT, led to an agreement to bring the subject before the next Quarterly meeting, with a view to the Yearly Meeting's proposing some sort of action against the trade.[17]

Quaker agitation continued and in 1881 a deputation from the Society of Friends was presented to the Secretary of State for India. But it was the Meeting for Sufferings' reports on the immorality of the opium traffic that were translated into positive action by the Quaker movement as a whole. The minutes and proceedings of the Yearly Meeting for 1880 recorded that:

> It has long been felt by many of our members to be a national sin thus to force a noxious and poisonous drug upon an unwilling nation . . . but be assured of the truth of the scripture declaration that it is righteousness which exalteth a nation, while sin is a reproach to any people, we would urge upon our rulers to do that which is just and right, confident that if that principle actuate our conduct as a nation, a blessing would attend it, and that apprehended difficulties would be overcome. We therefore conclude to prepare a Memorial to the Government on the subject to be presented by deputation of this meeting . . . The Meeting for Sufferings is also requested to give careful attention to the subject . . . for any further action upon it.[18]

QUAKER INFLUENCE ON SSOT STRUCTURE

The Society of Friends' structure was mirrored in the organisation of the SSOT and in doing so served two functions. First, it ensured recognition of the SSOT as a Quaker-like efficient business organisation which duly commanded and received pre-eminent respect within Victorian society. Second, and more significantly, it provided the means for organising within the SSOT an effective communications network. This network operated very simply. Missionaries, doctors, diplomats, journalists and so forth with experience, either at home or abroad, of those who took opium as a 'stimulant' would be invited to report it to local SSOT meetings up and down the country. These local reports were then compiled monthly for publication in *Friend of China*. At the Society's Annual General Meetings the overall picture portrayed by these reports was compiled. To the Quaker-dominated General Council these reports, which recurrently associated compulsive opium use with evidence of immorality, indicated the presence of a pathologically debilitated will.

What I have described then, are the conditions which both enabled the founders of the SSOT to know of addiction as a moral pathological phenomenon and for this idea to be taken seriously by those who were not Quakers and had nothing to do with the society. But this claim as to the cause of addiction did not just exist as an idea which the SSOT simply talked about. During the late nineteenth century the idea was used by others as if it were an object, in the same way that the idea of gravity, for example, has become used as an object which we refer to today when unblocking sinks, irrigating fields, distributing domestic water supplies and so forth. Quaker status and organisational structure therefore enabled the SSOT to talk about the idea of a moral pathological model of addiction. While they may be credited for its inception they did not 'discover' this model as a pre-formed object for presentation to the community. The transformation of their notion of addiction from that of an idea into a self-evident truth and thus endowed with the status of an object actually owed little to the SSOT itself. Instead a number of nineteenth-century institutions were implicated, some of which had little or no connection with Quakerism, the anti-opium movement or the development of the SSOT.

The common feature of all these institutions was their ability to distinguish, describe and discuss the SSOT's idea of a pathologically debilitated will as if it were a manifest, tangible object. In the conditions formed by these institutions it was possible to form a regime in which the truth of addiction was understood in this way. In the following chapter I offer a sample of these institutions, drawn from a much wider network, which during the late nineteenth century were capable of both taking this idea seriously and using it as a causal explanation for the compulsive use of opiates.

6 Forming the Moral Pathological Model as an Object

The potential for ideas is limited only by the human imagination. But the potential of these ideas to appear as, it were, as tangible objects is much more constrained. Although someone can say something new, for example 'homosexuality is a crime', in order for homosexuality to appear as a crime and a tangible object – comparable with or dissimilar to other objects of criminal action like theft – it has to be acknowledged within a complex group of social relations. The moral pathological model of addiction is a case in point. Although the idea clearly belonged to the SSOT's founders it was not simply their imagination alone which conditioned the existence of the model as a tangible object. Instead I argue that the object existed under the conditions of a complex group of social relations between late nineteenth-century institutions, three of which are explored; Literary Society, Medicine and Religion.

LITERARY SOCIETY AND MORAL PATHOLOGY

When De Quincey's *Confessions* were first serialised in 1821 public reaction was essentially 'a mixture of intelligent appreciation and sanctimonious condemnation'.[1] To a few, De Quincey's exaltations in praise of opium were nothing short of scandalous but, to many others, his reported experiences with opium were received with interest, excitement, even humour![2] The possibility that opium could be taken in order to stimulate the writer's imagination was an especially attractive thought in literary circles of the early to mid nineteenth century, at a time when the importance of the writer's imagination in providing a richness of style was increasingly appreciated and recognised. Appreciation of an opium-induced creative imagination was not confined to writers and artists alone. In recognition of this the *Medical Intelligencer*, a popular medical journal of the early nineteenth century, which was particularly impressed by De Quincey's 'beautiful narrative', was moved to advocate a wider usage of opium.[3] The *British Review*, however, cast a less positive light on De Quincey's revelations, arguing that it was 'not disposed to acquiesce in the justness of this panegyric of opium'.[4] While not sharing the *Medical Intelligencer's* view, the *Review* did not dispute in principle the possibility that opium could be conceived as a possible legitimate vehicle for facilitating creative writing. It simply did not agree with its use as a stimulant for creative productions.

By the end of the century however, this notion had significantly diminished in popularity both within and beyond the confines of literary society. In 1891 *Friend of China* reprinted an extract from the *Lancet* which reported that, 'in spite of the example set by Coleridge and De Quincey, the better sense of mankind has declared against habits which enslave both the mind and body and degrade the fine susceptibilities for the sake of transient exhilaration'.[5] The demise in popularity of taking opium as a creative stimulant was of course neither immediate nor absolute. During the Society of Arts debate on opium, held in 1892, there were those who, 'adduced De Quincey as commending the habit'.[6] Celebrations of opium's purported creative stimulant properties further continued into the following century with the publication of Aleister Crowley's *Diary of a Drug Fiend* in 1922 – exactly one hundred years after De Quincey's *Confessions* were first published in book form.

Crowley, the son of a wealthy 'scion of a race of Quakers'[7] was an enigmatic character with a considerable interest in the practice of magic and the occult. He died in 1947, a heroin addict, aged seventy-two but his controversial reputation extended beyond his death and he is to be found standing between an Indian holy man and Mae West in a composite photograph of 'People we like' on the sleeve of the Beatles' classic record of the 1960s, *Sgt Pepper's Lonely Hearts Club Band*. His acclaimed use of opiates as a stimulant for his literary writings enhanced his reputation. But he describes his initial experiences with opium as disappointing. While on a visit to Burma he had experimented with taking thirty grains of powdered opium, succeeding only in making himself, 'suddenly and painlessly sick'.[8] Passing through into China, he further experimented with smoking opium but found the experience equally unavailing. 'I smoked twenty-five pipes in five hours with no result whatever.'[9] His travels through China also left him sceptical of the claim that opium smoking was physically and morally debasing:

> During my whole journey, I never saw a man whom I could call definitely the worse for opium. My wife's chair coolies were cases in point. They had smoked from twelve years old or thereabout . . . Each man had to carry forty pounds . . . Each man had to keep in step with the rest and shake the chair as little as possible; and this over rough hilly roads, often slippery with mud; perhaps against a head wind, in which case the furniture of the chair offered a large surface. One of these coolies, the heaviest and most inveterate smoker of the quartet, cannot have been less than sixty years old. I timed the men under the worst conditions; a road mostly uphill, driving sleet – half a gale – dead ahead streaming slippery cobbles, and they did eight miles without a rest in two hours dead. If those were 'physical wrecks from the abuse of opium', I should like to see the animal in his undamaged state!'[10]

On leaving China he subsequently went on to appreciate opium's effects more fully while living in Paris. He recalls,

> I had a bad attack of influenza, which settled down to severe bronchitis. I was visited one evening by an old friend of mine and her young man, who very kindly and sensibly suggested I should find relief if I smoked a few pipes of opium. They accordingly brought the apparatus from their apartment and we began . . . My bronchitis vanished; I went off to sleep; my guests retiring without waking me. In my sleep I dreamt; and when I woke the dream remained absolutely perfect in my consciousness, down to the minutest detail. It was a story, a subtle exposure of English stupidity, set in a frame of the craziest and most fantastically gorgeous workmanship. Ill as I was, I jumped out of bed and wrote down the story offhand. I called it 'The Stratagem' [and] I was told – nothing in my life ever made me prouder – that Joseph Conrad said it was the best short story he had read in ten years.[11]

From the late nineteenth century onwards however, literary support for the practice of using opium as a creative stimulant had become very much an anachronistic exception rather than the rule. When De Quincey's *Confessions* were re-issued towards the end of the century – 13 editions and re-issues were published: more than in the first half of the century – it was by way of illustrating his habit as an issue of concern. This theme was taken up in the SSOT's journal *Friend of China*. In an 1890 issue it reported, 'No doubt it is a bad habit to take opium in any form or mode, a fact of which Coleridge and De Quincey, and more recently Wilkie Collins [author of the popular nineteenth-century detective novel, *The Moonstone*] have been melancholy and well known instances'.[12]

By the 1920s, literary society was similarly disdainful of Crowley and his opiate-induced writings. When *Diary of a Drug Fiend* appeared in November 1922 *The Times Literary Supplement* described it as 'a phantasmagoria of ecstacies, despairs and above all verbiage' and Crowley's works were otherwise largely ignored. James Douglas in his column in the Sunday Express described *The Diary of a Drug Fiend* as 'an ecstatic eulogy of the drug' and called for its suppression. Throughout the contemporary press of the 1920s Crowley was denounced as 'the most evil man in all of England'. Such scathing indictments were obviously directed solely against Crowley. His shaven head and hypnotic eyes coupled with his evil reputation, eccentric appearance and his passion for notoriety marked him out for public denouncement. What was at issue in the literary world however, was not Crowley's personal appearance but the worth of his 'drug-inspired' writings.

Between the first publication (in book form) of De Quincey's *Confessions* in 1822 and Crowley's *Confessions* one hundred years later, the criteria by which the production of literary work were gauged had changed. The use of opiates in order to stimulate a creative imagination had not simply fallen out of fashion. The legitimacy of such literary efforts could now be brought into question with the emerging authority of literary and art criticism. Literary work thus became treated less as a freely created object which could be judged simply in accordance with one's individual taste in creative forms (wherein opium could be legitimately considered as an important variable in assessing the worth of literary work), and more as the product of a skilled exercise. Literary creations then were to be judged by deciphering within them the authors' own skills. The knowledge which constituted literary skills had become codified and in the process literary society's concept of opium as a creative stimulant had become redundant. There was no place in the disciplined exercise of creativity for literary objects that were produced by dint of some opium-induced, unstructured blind inspiration.

By the late nineteenth century then patrons of literary society had virtually ceased to offer their own account and explanation of opium's effects as a creative stimulant. Against their silence which served to acknowledge what the opium habit was *not*, i.e. a legitimate aid to creative imagination, emerged positive testimonies by other communities of the moral-pathological basis of opiate dependence. During the late nineteenth century the medical profession could be included among those who identified the cause of compulsive opium use in a pathologically debilitated will.

MEDICINE AND MORAL PATHOLOGY

Medical concern with opium for much of the nineteenth century focused on the debate as to whether opium acted as a stimulant or sedative on the habitué's nervous system. The 'opium habit' was discussed among doctors as an object which was understood as a collection of pharmacological properties. Although opium's addictive qualities had been known for centuries the phenomenon of dependence remained a medical curiosity for much of the century, possibly because the bulk of opium was consumed in England in proprietary form, primarily for self-medication. Observations reported in the *Friend of China*, that the English 'generally have no immediate experience . . . of opium eating or smoking',[13] reflected the novelty of addiction for doctors, and the overall lack of attention paid to the addicted state. Seven years later, in contrast, *Friend of China* reported: 'Many are aware that this drug has been used non-medically in many parts of the country, to the great injury, physically and morally, of numerous individuals'.[14] None had become more aware of this than the doctors themselves. By the late nineteenth century, in medical discourse, the compulsive use of opium was no longer described as an individual's relatively innocuous habit.

Failed attempts to find a physiological basis for addiction[15] which had previously sustained the medical understanding of the habit as comprising the observed stimulant/sedative effect was replaced by a description of the compulsive use of opiates which doctors could refer to as a 'moral pathological' phenomenon. At the SSOT's Annual General Meeting of 1886, Dr Foster argued that opium, 'saps the moral nature, deteriorates the moral character, and one loses all sense of moral obligation'. Medical language described not just the effects of the habit but also analysed its cause in terms of a pathologised moral faculty.

Medical treatment for those who had developed the dependence syndrome clearly underlined this thinking. An 1877 issue of the *Lancet* reported in its editorial the belief that morphia addiction degraded the moral character and advocated that, 'Moral treatment by urging them early to some form of steady work, is particularly to be insisted upon'.[16] Towards the end of the century this concept of a pathologically debilitated will as an explanation of the aetiology of compulsive opiate use was popular among doctors. Dr William Huntley argued that 'the longer the habit is continued, the more the willpower is abolished, the moral judgement weakened'.[17] Some doctors further sought to clearly distinguish the medically established physiological effects of opium from its effect on the moral faculty. During a House of Commons debate in 1875 on the Opium Trade, the Rev. R. H. Graves, a medically qualified missionary, differentiated the physiological effects of opium (stimulating the nervous system) from its social and moral effects (inciting lethargy).

Similar accounts defining compulsive opiate use in physiological terms and by extension as a medical phenomenon proliferated during the late nineteenth century. For example, an 'Important Medical Declaration' in an 1892 issue of *Friend of China* noted 5230 medical men practising in Great Britain signed a declaration stating that, 'the habit of opium smoking, or of opium eating, is morally and physically debasing'.[18] None the less medical accounts ultimately located its aetiology in the individual's will or moral faculty: a point substantiated in a supplement to *Friend of China* entitled, 'The Medical Aspect of the Opium Question'.[19] They could do so by acknowledging the notion of a metaphorical material soul – a distinctive Quaker object – containing a moral faculty whose health or ill-health, development or retardation could be analysed in material terms, as an affiliated medical object. At issue here is the possibility that medicine could register the SSOT's model of addiction as a 'normal' medical object to be discussed among doctors just as they might discuss a fracture or an infection.

RELIGION AND MORAL PATHOLOGY

The slight moral protestations resulting from De Quincey's revelations were uncoordinated and reflected a notable absence of institutionalised concern over gratuitous opium consumption in Britain. Fears voiced about the immoral consequences following non-medical use of opium were based largely on reports from missionaries returning from overseas. Overall, within both the orthodox and non-conformist religious communities, revelations of a self-confessed opium habit of a British citizen did not appear to register as an invariant evil. That is, compulsive use of opium was not considered to be an issue which fell within their frame of concern. However, by the late nineteenth century this 'conceptual threshold' had shifted such that it was possible to incorporate within it a range of concepts which had belonged to and were previously used exclusively by Quakers. Whereas the religious community's piecemeal anti-opium stance had previously consisted of an automatic response against vice throughout much of the Victorian era, by the late nineteenth century their opposition to opium was underscored by a new comprehension of dependence. Key elements of this new comprehension included the concept of a moral faculty of the soul that could be pathologised, and the possibility of establishing in certain material practices an intrinsic correspondence with the state of one's moral faculty. Within this new conceptual threshold the opium habit became apprehended by religion-inspired moralists in terms of a pathologically debilitated moral faculty.

Evidence of this new threshold dates back to the 1880s when conformist and non-conformist religious sects sought to identify and associate with the SSOT's aims and objectives. In 1881 a public meeting to discuss the opium trade was organised by the SSOT. It was held in London's Mansion House and chaired by the Lord Mayor. Significantly his two chief supporters on the platform were both clergymen; the Archbishop of Canterbury and a Cardinal Manning. By 1886 an editorial in *Friend of China* boasted, 'There is not an assembly of a Christian church which did not back us in our efforts by their petitions and memorials'.[20] J. W. Pease himself was given to exhort 'We have the churches all with us in a most remarkable way. We have presented to the House of Commons a petition signed by every Roman Catholic dignitary in the United Kingdom. I presented a petition which was signed by all the bishops of the Church of England, I think without exception. We have had petitions from the convocations of north and south, petitions from all the convocations of the religious bodies in the United Kingdom.'[21]

Further evidence of wider conformist and non-conformist involvement in the Society emerged as the century progressed. An anti-opium meeting was organised by the Society in 1890, at Newcastle-upon-Tyne, under the chairmanship of the Lord Bishop of the Diocese, the Rt Rev. Dr E. Wilberforce.[22] In the same year, the Mayor of Sunderland was moved to observe at another anti-opium meeting that he was glad to think there were gentlemen of all religious creeds present.[23] Support by conformist religions continued: in the following year, at the SSOT's annual general meeting, the Society's president, Joseph Whitwell Pease was supported on the platform by the Venerable Archdeacon Moule and the Rev. Wilberforce. By 1897, the Society was able to count among its vice presidents five Anglican Bishops.[24]

The final decade of the nineteenth century also saw increasing support from the non-conformist sects. In 1890, at the Autumn Conference of the Quaker's Evangelical Alliance, and before the Presbytery of the Edinburgh United Presbyterian Church, resolutions supporting the SSOT were passed unanimously. Non-conformists could also be counted on the Society's General Council.[25] By 1892, representatives from the Baptist church, the Wesleyan church, the Primitive Methodists, Congregation Unionist Church, the Free Church of Scotland and the United Methodist Free Church could all be found supporting the SSOT's cause.[26]

Six years later, the Presbyterian Church of England, the Calvinistic Methodists of Wales, and the General Body of Protestant dissenting ministers were added to the 'long list of Christian Churches' who protested against opium.

CONCLUDING COMMENTS

In the early nineteenth century medical practice, literary society and the religious community viewed the issue of opium use in different ways. At issue for medicine was opium's psychopharmacological properties, i.e. whether opium acted as a sedative or stimulant on the nervous system. Patrons of literary society conceived opium as a legitimate vehicle to stimulate in writers a creative imagination. Within the religious community its effects indicated its non-medical use as a vice. Clearly medicine could also view it as a vice too, just as literary society could not dismiss opium's sedative effect, but the interpretation each community gave of these effects differed significantly from the others'.

Yet by the late nineteenth century the effects of opium could be commonly understood, either directly or by implication, in terms of a pathologically debilitated moral faculty. In the intervening years what had been to all intent and purpose nothing more than an idea belonging to a group of Quaker social reformers, emerged with the status of a palpable and widely accepted object. The medical, literary and religious communities, among others, played a significant role in this process. Between them they mapped out a space in which this idea was singled out, talked about, taken seriously and used as if it were an object. These communities however, are not arbitrarily selected. They have been identified for their specific qualities which include, among others, their capacity to exercise their own brand of authoritative judgement on the effects of opium which acknowledges, testifies to and 'normalises' it as an object. I have identified three such judgements; literary, religious and medical, but there are undoubtedly more.

It was therefore in the space of the relations between these communities that the Quaker model of addiction existed, not just as an idea but one which could be used as an object. But it did not exist alone. Throughout the period during which SSOT promulgated the moral pathological model, medical specialists on addiction made a counter-claim that addiction was in fact a disease which afflicted the individual's will. But reformulating the concept of addiction as a new object, i.e. a disease, depends on new prevailing conditions which could give rise to the possibility of its existence. In the following chapter, the claims of these addiction specialists are examined to show that if they constituted addiction as a new object.

7 From Moral Illness to Pathological Disease

Johnson[1] has suggested that the activities of the SSOT correspond broadly to those of what Becker terms 'moral entrepreneurs'. According to Becker there are two species of 'moral entrepreneurs', rule creators and rule enforcers. In that the founders of the SSOT present a classic example of the rule creator, it is worth quoting Becker's definition at length.

> A rule creator, . . . is interested in the content of rules. The existing rules do not satisfy him because there is some evil which profoundly disturbs him. He feels that nothing can be right in the world until rules are made to correct it. He operates with an absolute ethic; what he sees is truly and totally evil with no qualification. Any means is justified to do away with it. The crusader is fervent and righteous, often self-righteous. It is appropriate to think of reformers as crusaders because they typically believe that their mission is a holy one. The prohibitionist serves as an excellent example, as does the person who wants to suppress vice and sexual delinquency or the person who wants to do away with gambling. These examples suggest that the moral crusader is a meddling busybody, interested in forcing his own morals on others. But this is a one-sided view. Many moral crusaders have strong humanitarian overtones. The crusader is not only interested in seeing to it that other people do what he thinks right. He believes that if they do what is right it will be good for them.[2]

The founders of the SSOT would indeed appear to be 'moral entrepreneurs'. They ruled that the opium trade with China was immoral because the drug was being consumed not for medical purposes but merely as an intoxicant which debilitated one's moral faculty. However, they differed from Becker's definition in at least one significant respect. Becker states that moral crusaders would frequently rely on the advice of experts when drawing up their lines of campaign. During the SSOT's campaign it was the support of experts for the testimonies of the morally debilitating effects of opium which was sought rather than expert advice on the nature and cause of addiction. Each issue of *Friend of China* contained numerous medical references testifying to both the physiological and spiritually debilitating effects of opium. These were consolidated in a supplement accompanying a 1892 issue which was entitled 'The Medical Aspects of the Opium Question'. The supplement contained testimonies of the physical and moral effects of opium gathered from doctors and medical missionaries who had direct experience of working with opium addicts both at home and abroad. This medical evidence provided a forceful counterbalance against claims by those who were pro-opium (including a small number of doctors) who argued that opium, and therefore its trade, was not in fact harmful.

Before the formation of the SSOT, however, a group of doctors had already proposed a model of addiction which strongly contrasted with the moral pathological model. Instead of locating the cause of addiction in a debilitated will, they argued addiction was defined as a disease which, like any other medically defined disease, had a physical cause. A growing number of doctors who began to specialise in addiction towards the end of the nineteenth century helped to further refine this 'medical' model. Undoubtedly the growth and development of medical interest and the emergence of addiction as a medical specialist area, complete with its own 'experts', contributed significantly to compounding medicine's authority on the subject. But what these 'experts' proposed was in fact a reformulated moral pathological model.

MEDICINE AND MORPHIA

Until well into the 1860s medical interest in opiates was concerned primarily with whether they acted as a stimulant or a sedative on the habitué's nervous system. Although attempts had been made during the first half of the nineteenth century to locate a physical cause of addiction these had failed.[3] The growing popularity of a stronger opiate than opium together with new methods of administering it however provided a new issue of interest for medicine. From the 1870s onwards in Great Britain, the focus of medical concern over opiates shifted to morphine and the nature of its administration. Its subcutaneous injection by hypodermic syringe, usually for the management of pain, was a favoured practice among doctors in General Practice and hospitals because of its effective speed of action and relatively small dosage required. This development gave a focus for the enquiries of the newly emergent addiction specialists. Among the first in Great Britain to draw attention to the potential dangers of injecting morphine was Dr Thomas Clifford Allbutt. On becoming aware that his regular morphine using patients were presenting similar symptoms, he suggested that repeated doses of morphine might have attendant dangers.[4]

Edward Levinstein, a German psychiatrist, provided perhaps the most significant contribution to medical specialist addiction literature during the 1870s with the publication in 1877 of *Die Morphiumsucht*, translated the following year into English as *Morbid Cravings for Morphia*. The text had all the hallmarks of a dispassionate medical study, with sections dealing with symptoms, cause and prognosis of dependence on morphia. More importantly, it ruled out the possibility that addiction was of psychosomatic origin. In describing morphia addiction as 'the uncontrollable desire of a person to use morphia as a stimulant and a tonic, and a diseased state of the system caused by the injudicious use of the said remedy',[5] Levinstein wished to distinguish morphia addiction not as a state of mental or moral alienation, but as a pathological morbid craving. The desire for morphia injections, he stressed, resulted from a person's natural constitution and not, as in the case of the 'moral pathological' model, from a certain predisposition to its use.[6] Opiate addiction which had previously been considered at best a bad habit, and at worst an immoral state, was reformulated by Levinstein as a morbid pathological disease.

In proposing addiction to have a physical cause and which required the attention of a physician, Levinstein clearly envisaged treatment to be a medical rather than a moral issue. However despite this the core of Levinstein's treatment programme underscored a perception not, as with other medical issues, of a pathological disease which was located in the internal organs of the body, but instead of a debilitated will. What Levinstein sought to treat was not some morbid lesion which caused the compulsion for morphia but instead the symptoms. These manifested themselves as the addict's inability to resist the morphia-induced cravings. Treatment therefore was concerned primarily with bolstering up the patient's moral reserves by means of re-educating the addict's will. Failure to affect a cure was therefore in the final analysis an individual responsibility.

ADDICTION AS A 'DISEASE OF THE WILL'

In Britain perhaps the most significant medical spokesman on addiction during the nineteenth century was Dr Norman Kerr. In 1884, Kerr founded and presided over the Society for the Study of Inebriety (SSI) – an association of eminent medical men whose task was: 'to investigate the various causes of inebriety and to educate the professional and public mind to a recognition of the physical aspects of intemperance.'[7]

Although Kerr's primary concern was with alcohol consumption, he did write about 'narcotising agents', which included opiates. Deliberations within the SSI had given rise, by the 1880s, to a psychosomatic theory of addiction based on the assumption that 'inebriety had its origin in vice and its seat in the brain'.[8] This assumption was applied to opiate addiction in 1887 with the publication of Kerr's *Inebriety or Narcomania*. In it he sought to establish addiction not as a willful act but a diseased state, thereby explaining in pathological terms why it was that some people continued to give in to their cravings although they remained aware of the probable consequences to their health. He conceded this state rarely exhibited organic lesions, arguing instead that it was a functional neurosis, i.e. addiction being resultant on a mentally defective state which had its source in localised brain lesions. Kerr posited the existence of a metabolic or structural anomaly – a diathesis – which explained the most characteristic feature of the disease: the inability to resist a compulsive craving for opiates. This did not represent to Kerr a stage in the victim's sinfulness but the developed stage of a disease, the point at which 'there is a departure from health in the form of some obscure condition of the nervous system, which craves for the temporary relief afforded by some stimulant or narcotic'.[9] The diathesis, according to Kerr, was a sort of pathological triggering mechanism that could be provoked into action by the repeated intoxication from opiates. The malnutrition of the cerebral and nerve tissue caused by such dosages led to an impairment of the inhibitory process located in the brain. For Kerr, addiction was a disease whose characteristic symptoms he described as, 'an overpowering impulse to indulge in intoxication at all risks.'[10] Having interpreted these symptoms, they indicated to Kerr the advanced stages of mental and moral decay. 'Opium', Kerr argued, 'is a poison which excites, intoxicates and enervates the whole man; by repeated indulgence inducing bodily and mental prostrations and moral perversions.'[11]

The cause of addiction however was taken to be physical although no physical causation had been demonstrated to exist from pathological explorations. Kerr however was adamant that a pathological site within the body caused the addiction: 'of its existence', he maintained, 'I do not see how there can be any reasonable doubt'.[12]

By the late nineteenth century the SSI, with Kerr as its figure-head, had publicised in some British medical circles the idea that opiate addiction was a disease. Addiction therefore warranted medical treatment. The form this treatment took however was based on the same perception of addiction which Levinstein had articulated in the previous decade. Essentially Kerr advocated a three-stage treatment programme. First, withdrawal of the drug; second, the removal of the precipitating cause of the drug's use; and finally, the repair of any physical damage. The treatment called for strict environmental control, preferably within the confines of an institution – an asylum or nursing home – on the rationale that they provided 'everything which can contribute to the improvement of the soul and the spirit, as well as to the reparative of tissue'.[13]

The underlying notion of treating morphia-addicted patients for a lapsed will was also evident in Oscar Jennings' celebrated treatment of 'voluntary withdrawal'. Like Kerr, Jennings was equally adamant that addiction was not a mere vice but a disease with a physical cause, a point made unequivocally in the preface of *The Re-Education of Self-Control in the Treatment of the Morphia Habit (1909)*: 'The moral obliquity of mankind does not come within the range of materia medica'.[14]

Morphia habitués, he maintained, were not willing victims of the drug but sick people whose 'will had laid dormant' because of a 'psychosomatic affection'. But neither was the craving for morphia a pathological entity, 'like malaria or syphilis and curable by agents like quinine, atoxyl or mercury, acting on a *materies morbi*, but a general pathological disturbance caused by the withdrawal of an accustomed stimulant which affects all the functions of the body'.[15] Treatment was therefore oriented towards restoring the patient's will in order to resist the craving. To do so Jennings insisted on a condition of 'moral hygiene' whereby relatives of the patient would refrain from being 'impatient, quarrelous, discouraging or reproachful.'

By nature the morphia-dependent patient Jennings described is 'tenacious of discouragement'. Voluntary withdrawal therefore involved removing from the patient's mind the image of the 'distressing moral cause' of the morphia dependence, in order to build up sufficient 'moral energy' to sustain the patient through the period of withdrawal. 'Moral orthopaedics' or the 're-education of the emotivity' was central to Jenning's treatment: 'One has the health of one's character; if the character is improved the health improves also. The patient must then be encouraged progressively, and taught at first to put up as courageously as possible with little discomforts and little discouragements. The will is weak because the power is weakened.'[16] Resolute confidence, then, was the keynote to the successful management of morphia addicts not just of the patient but, Jennings added, of the doctor in his conviction of his own ability to help!

Jennings was also opposed to the practice of attempting to wean patients off morphia by substituting in its place alcohol or even heroin. Although this was already gaining popularity among some 'specialists', he declared especially of the use of heroin that 'to prescribe a still stronger narcotic stimulant, in a disease of the will, characterised by post-stimulant hyper-irritability, is not logical'.[17] Instead he proposed a regimen of a progressively diminishing quantity of morphia in a solution of salt. When the daily dose had been reduced to 2 grains a day injections should be given, not in the arm but in the rectum. For those who had developed chronic dependence – 'drug fiends' who could not be treated at home – they would require treatment in a special drug sanatorium.

The distinction between those who were merely dependent on morphia and those whose dependence resembled that of a mania (Jennings used the term 'narcomania') was also drawn by an American physician, Dr T. D. Crothers. He distinguished morphinism and morphinomania. Morphinism describes 'a condition following the prolonged use of morphin (sic)', while morphinomania is designated, 'the condition of persons in whom the impulse to use morphin, is the nature of a mania, possessing the mind and dominating every thought, leaving but one supreme desire – to procure morphin and experience the pleasure it gives.'[18] The morphinist, having contracted the habit, was held to have retained his moral sensibilities and sanity and thereby wished to be cured; while the morphinomaniac had lost both and was irredeemably addicted. This distinction was taken up in England and sensationalised by newspaper reports of so-called morphinomaniacs whose addiction had led them to commit murder. Among them the Lawson case is particularly notable in that it caused an immense sensation.

Lawson, an American doctor, had been in the habit of taking opium in the form of cigarettes, the tobacco being impregnated with opium, since serving as a young medical attendant during the siege of Paris. On being discharged for dispensing opium cigarettes to wounded soldiers, Lawson returned to America where he went on from the use of opium cigarettes to larger and larger quantities of morphine. Following a number of failed attempts in the United States to rid himself of the habit he came to England where he obtained money to live on and buy his opium by forging cheques. Finally, in 1882, he was convicted and condemned to death for the murder of his brother-in-law, on whose death Lawson would have been entitled to one thousand five hundred pounds. Despite attempts by the President of the United States, Secretary of State for the USA, and a large number of American doctors, bishops and clergymen to obtain a reprieve for Lawson on the grounds that he was a 'morphio-maniac', the unfortunate doctor was duly hanged at Wandsworth Gaol, London, on 28 April 1882.

A similar fate befell another addicted doctor. Dr Neill was convicted of murdering six women with the idea of blackmailing his acquaintances with false charges of murder. At his trial, evidence testifying to the fact that Neill was an 'opium slave' was offered. In the United States, perhaps, such evidence might have provided for a plea of mitigating circumstances for his actions on the grounds that he was a morphinomaniac, but in late nineteenth-century England it was damning evidence and Neill was hanged for his crimes in Newgate prison on 15 November 1892.

By now the idea of a morphinomaniac had captured the public's imagination. Writing on morphine addiction in the popular journal, *Nineteenth Century*, in 1887, Seymour Sharkey noted that such terms as morphinomania indicated, 'an uncontrollable craving for morphia which is said to be demoralising an ever-increasing number of people in this and other countries'.[19] Sainsbury, another specialist, called addiction a form of moral insanity,[20] while Sir William Collins popularised Jennings' notion of a 'disease of the will'.

By the turn of the twentieth century these medical specialists offered a theory of the cause of addiction which, unlike the 'moral pathological model', extolled scientific respectability with its emphasis on biological determinism. But in many respects there was little to commend this medical model over that of the SSOT.

Opiates were presumed to affect the body physically, primarily through their actions on the brain and central nervous system. These effects were expressed behaviourally as a craving. Treatment therefore operated on two fronts. First the opiate which had induced the behaviour was reduced or terminated. Second, having removed or at least regulated the consumption of the drug which had initiated the craving, these specialists sought to treat the addicts' continued craving for morphia, not as an organic physical problem, but a behavioural one. The way in which these specialists perceived this behavioural problem and hence the way in which they responded to it would appear to correspond to the SSOT's perception of addiction.

Psychologically-determined behavioural problems today are distinguished from other types of problems in that they can be established empirically, using experimental techniques which control for variables such as personality type, family background and so forth. Such behavioural problems are not of a generic type but classified into certain categories in accordance with these variables. These addiction specialists, however, did not classify the behavioural problem of the morphia addicted patient empirically. Instead, they reasoned it to be a generically moral problem involving one's 'will'. To resist their craving required strong willpower. Failure to do so in every instance commensurately indicated a lack of willpower.[21] Treatment therefore was designed to restore the patients' morally debilitated 'will' so that they could renounce their addiction.

At issue here is the fact that these specialists could exercise a judgement on addiction as a behavioural problem which was classified within a framework of moral rather than definitively medical judgements. Moreover, despite the specialists' emphasis on a biological cause of addiction as a 'disease of the will', these moral judgements on which their prescribed treatment was based, appeared to replicate those exercised by the SSOT in constructing the 'moral pathological' model. In terms of providing an understanding of the cause of addiction, these models were interchangeable. Both were constructed using reason alone rather than empirical techniques; both considered addiction a generic behavioural problem concerning the moral faculty; and both emphasised the moral charge of addiction as ultimately an individual problem.

However, by the second decade of the present century, medical references to addiction as a 'disease of the will' had become obsolete. Although doctors continued to treat addicts in much the same way they had done in the past, the thinking behind treatment had changed. Gradually diminishing doses of opiates were no longer administered as an interim measure to deal with the main behavioural problem of the addict's lost willpower. Doctors did not aim at restoring the addict's willpower, but restoring the addict's physical health. They therefore sought to treat the patient's dependence on opiates not as a function of a loss of willpower but as a function of a pathological disease whose symptoms according to medical judgement had no bearing on one's moral status or strength of will. Medical rather than moral judgement, then, formed the basis for this treatment. This judgement was founded on medicine's understanding of the effects of disease on the body's pathological functioning. Dependence on opiates altered this functioning but abrupt withdrawal could compromise it further, possibly leading to its complete collapse and the addict's death. Regular, diminishing doses therefore served to help gradually restore the addict's diseased body back to normal functioning. The treatment of addiction had by the 1920s become a medical issue based on a definitively medical judgement.

ADDICTION AS A PATHOLOGICAL DISEASE

The emergence of addiction as a definitively medical object was preceded by attempts to establish the regulation of narcotics as a matter of social policy. The first legislative measures against narcotics were not taken until the second decade of the present century, and were then instigated under conditions peculiar to war-time.[22] The 1916 Defence of the Realm Act Regulation 40B restricted both the sale and possession of cocaine and opium. Underlying this regulation was a penal response which was developed further in subsequent legislation. The 1920 Dangerous Drugs Act extended the 1916 restrictions to cover morphine as well as cocaine and opium. Further Home Office regulations made under the Act, in 1921 and 1922,[23] underscored a predominately prohibitionist policy that had already matured in the USA.[24]

But the case for medical control of addiction – on the grounds it was a medically defined pathological disease – was already being formulated in Great Britain amidst ambiguities in the Act, as to whether 'treatment' for addiction could be regarded as legitimate medical practice or not. In order to clarify the issue, the then Ministry of Health appointed a Departmental Committee in 1924. The Committee, chaired by Sir Humphrey Rolleston, President of the Royal College of Physicians and Regius Professor of Physics at Cambridge, was composed entirely of medical men. Its terms of reference were specific: 'to consider and advise as to the circumstances, if any, in which the supply of morphine and heroin (including preparations containing morphine and heroin) to persons suffering from addiction to those drugs may be regarded as medically advisable, and as to the precautions which it is desirable that medical practitioners administering or prescribing morphine or heroin should adopt for the avoidance of abuse'.[25]

The Committee took evidence almost exclusively from medical witnesses and reported its findings in 1926. The addict, it recommended, be defined as: 'a person who, not requiring the continued use of the drug for the relief of the symptoms of organic disease has acquired, as a result of repeated administration, an overpowering desire for its continuance, and in whom withdrawal of the drug leads to definite symptoms of mental or physical distress or disorder.'[26] The report's central recommendation was that two classes of person should continue to be maintained on non-decreasing doses of opiates: 'Those in whom a complete withdrawal of morphine or heroin produces serious symptoms which cannot be treated satisfactorily under the normal conditions of private practice, and those who are capable of leading a fairly normal and useful life so long as they take a certain quantity, usually small, of their drug of addiction, but not otherwise'.[27]

The Committee concluded that heroin and morphine could be prescribed to certain addicts as 'legitimate medical treatment' but only under certain conditions and for certain classes of patients, namely:

(a) Those who are undergoing treatment for the cure of addiction by gradual withdrawal;
(b) Persons for whom, after every effort has been made for the cure of addiction, the drug cannot be completely withdrawn either because (i) Complete withdrawal produces serious symptoms which cannot be satisfactorily treated under the ordinary conditions of private practice; or (ii) The patient, while capable of leading a useful life so long as he takes a certain non-progressive quantity, usually small, of the drug of addiction, ceases to be able to do so when the regular allowance is withdrawn.

The report affirmed the disease model of addiction in which the addict is portrayed as a victim of a morbid and overpowering craving and whose diseased state required medical attention.

The Committee's recommendations were accepted by the Home Office and it was agreed that doctors would be allowed, in certain circumstances, to prescribe heroin and morphine to addicted patients: an agreement which formed the basis of the 'British System' for dealing with drug addiction. But the Home Office was prepared to endorse the Committee's recommendations only so long as it considered the medical profession's control to be effective. Drug policy thus remained subject to penal legislation, with unauthorised possession of dangerous drugs without a prescription sanctioned against in criminal law. Although doctors staked a claim to define the nature and treatment of addiction in accordance with definitively medical judgements, drug policy and its administration remained a Home Office matter.[28]

None the less doctors had succeeded in getting their judgement on the nature and causation of addiction as a disease accepted as the basis for a distinctive treatment policy. However, a central feature of this policy – the recommendation that doctors be allowed to prescribe a non-diminishing opiate dosage to addicts – was not new. As early as 1857, in evidence to the Select Committee on the Sale of Poisons Bill, Professor Alfred Taylor suggested that confirmed users be given a six month certificate to pick up their drug supply from a chemist.[29] Levinstein had similarly proposed that addicts be given a small quantity of an opiate if they were in danger of collapse, and Taylor's recommendations were again echoed by Crothers in 1902.[30] Although the 'Rolleston Report' (as it came to be known) was partly a re-affirmation of a previously-ignored recommendation, there was a fundamental difference in the thinking behind the Rolleston Committee's recommendations on addiction which set it apart from earlier similar recommendations.

The difference did not lie in the prescription itself – that addicts be given a non-diminishing dose of opiate – but lay instead in the basis of the doctors' medical knowledge from which they were able to judge this as proper medical treatment for addiction. The earlier prescriptions of Taylor and Crothers were based on an understanding of the addict as sick, but the thinking behind their recommendation for prescribing maintenance doses was not any different from that which enabled other medical specialists to talk of addiction as a disease of the will. Although the recommendation that established addicts be maintained on opiates appeared to indicate an attempt to treat addiction not as a behavioural issue involving a lapsed will, but as an organic disease, the basis for this judgement was the same. That is, doctors had made sense of addiction and how best to treat it by using only their ability for intuitive reasoning. The prevalent medical approach to addiction which primarily involved restoring the addict's debilitated will was founded on this basis. The practice of prescribing non-diminishing doses of opiates which continually debilitated the addict's willpower undermined this prevalent approach and there were no new grounds on which to challenge the dominant medical view of addiction as a disease of the will and make out a case that addiction was an organic disease requiring maintenance doses. In accordance with the nature of late nineteenth-century medical enquiries in addiction, to sustain an organic disease model of addiction for which maintenance doses could be prescribed would reasonably and logically require there to be an organic source to which medical treatment could be directed. As no such source had been located the possibility of putting forward the notion of an organic medical model was untenable and therefore not a real option.

By 1926 however, following the Rolleston Committee's recommendations, the principle of maintenance dose prescribing had become enshrined in the Dangerous Drugs Acts of the 1920s and was subsequently incorporated into medical orthodoxy, yet no organic site for addiction had been located. A major change in the nature of medical judgements facilitated this development. Intuition alone no longer provided the basis for judging addiction as a disease for which maintenance doses could be given. The

Rolleston Report's recommendations were made in accordance with a new form of medical judgement in which ideas founded on intuitive reasoning and devoid of any empirical substance played a much smaller part.

Treatment for addiction was prescribed for the first time in accordance with a judgement which only doctors were capable of making. This was a *clinical* judgement; a scientific judgement based on empirical techniques rather than on powers of reason alone. A feature of this exclusively medical judgement is that it is made on the basis of a particular understanding of how the living body functioned and how it becomes compromised by the actions of a disease. In accordance with their understanding doctors could make a clinical judgement defining addiction as a pathological disease purely on the basis of its effects on the functioning of the body and not (as with the earlier efforts of Kerr and his associates) by establishing its pathological source in some diseased organ.

The incorporation into medical orthodoxy of addiction as a pathological disease which could be treated with prescriptions for maintenance doses of opiates had nothing to do with a developed understanding of its cause – no organic source of addiction had been discovered. Instead the significant development concerned the ability of doctors to cast a new and distinctly medical judgement on addiction in the 1920s. Passing a clinical judgement on the addicted state then provided the basis for a definitively medical service for addicts that was to continue unchanged in Great Britain for over four decades. In the following chapter I shall suggest how it was possible for doctors to make this crucially important judgement which defined addiction as a pathologically diseased state without reference to the source of the disease in some organ of the body.

8 Pathology and the Medical Model

The Rolleston Report broke new ground with its concept of the addict as sick and addiction as a pathological disease, characterised by a 'morbid' craving for the drug. In order to fully appreciate the concept of disease, it is first necessary to understand the development of the contemporary view of 'disease' as such.

THE RISE OF SCIENTIFIC MEDICINE

The exercise of clinical judgements by doctors based on scientific principles as distinct from non-clinical judgements founded on empirically uninformed intuitive reason is a feature of a unified medical profession. This unity is however comparatively recent. The origins of organised medical care in England date back to 1518 when the Royal College of Physicians of London was founded.[1] The College was instituted to regulate the teaching and supply of physicians in the area of London. It held a monopoly over the regulation of the practice of 'physic' and its privileged members constituted a distinctive social group, sharing a common university education at Oxbridge.

Other branches of medical services such as surgeons and apothecaries did not enjoy a commensurate status. Up until 1745 surgeons and barbers were joined in a craft guild – 'Surgeon-Barbers Company of the City of London' – and it was not until 1800 that surgeons received their independence with the granting of a charter for the 'Royal College of Surgeons'.

The Apothecaries Act of 1815 served to consolidate this sectarian practice of medical care by legitimating the apothecary's practice of compounding and selling drugs. Greater accessibility of the apothecaries to the mass population and the failure of physicians to prescribe and meet the needs of the less affluent population led to greater reliance on these medical attendants.[2]

The medical services available in the first part of the nineteenth century consisted of distinctly organised, segregated and legally defined status groups. Physicians practicing the 'art of physic', surgeons the 'craft' of surgery, and apothecaries their 'trade'. Any consensus of values and norms among nineteenth-century medical attendants was therefore unlikely given their heterogeneous social backgrounds. Until 1858, medical services were hierarchically organised: segregated by class, wealth and education, which regulated access to the various medical fields though there were numerous attempts at reforming the practice of medicine along more unified lines during the nineteenth century. A most vociferous critic of this tripartite system and ardent agitator for reform was Thomas Wakley, who founded the 'Lancet' in 1823. An influential spokesman, he campaigned ceaselessly for reform of the system, claiming it was monopolistic and conspiratorial and therefore ran contrary to the interests of the general public and the ordinary practitioner.

The failure to unify medicine into a professional structure during the early nineteenth century indicated the general public's doubting attitude towards medicine: a medicine which was defined and practised often in the ambiguous context of 'quack' competition and too frequently oriented to the values, tastes and whims of affluent patients. As late as 1850 there were still

> those forming the utterly respectable supporters of the 'Ministry', and who believed in the orthodox practitioners; who have faith in the Royal College of Physicians and Surgeons and the Worshipful Society of Apothecaries; believe in fever, inflammation, boils, gout, consumption and other maladies; who call things by old names . . .; send for the doctor just as soon as they are ill, do exactly as they are bid, inquire simply whether the liver is affected or the head, and are satisfied with what they term his 'pronouncings' . . . they respect most highly someone who knows their constitution; and who knew their fathers . . . they believe in bilious attacks, and giving themselves up to the man who brought them into the world or sent their fathers out, they are bothered with no doubts, and are content to be killed or cured in the orthodox way.[3]

The culturally sanctioned working-class practice of self-medication and the publication of numerous journals during the nineteenth century which provided cheap and accessible homeopathic remedies for ailments, ensured that medical practice began more often in the home with little dependence on practitioners.[4]

By the early twentieth century, the sectarian organisation of medicine into physicians, surgeons and apothecaries had given way to a unified medical profession. Central to this unity was a corpus of medical knowledge which included an understanding of the pathological basis of disease. The clinical judgement is therefore founded on a uniquely medical understanding of the principles of pathological functioning. Applying these principles it was possible for doctors to establish the aetiology of a diseased pathological state for which no pathological source, i.e. a diseased organ in the body, could be found.

The development of these principles was made possible by a particular medical technique. Foucault, in his seminal work *Birth of the Clinic*,[5] terms this technique the *gaze*. It is a technique used by doctors to decipher the signs of disease on the visible body in order to reveal the state of the body's pathological functioning of the internal organs which lay beneath, without having to first dissect it. The doctor's clinical judgement is founded on an ability to view the body as if it were transparent, therefore allowing the aetiology of a disease to be localised either in some organ or more broadly within the body as a pathological state. In either case responsibility for the definition of disease remains exclusively that of the medical profession because of the scientific basis of their clinical judgement. How then was this medical vision of pathological functioning which was so crucial to the medical definition of addiction as a disease possible?

THE PRINCIPLES OF METAPHYSICAL PATHOLOGIES

Until the mid-1800s British medical practice would frequently involve an uncritical acceptance of traditional medical dogma and theories by both physician and patient alike, together with the swingeing use of treatments and heroic remedies which had been in vogue from the time of the first medical practitioners – the priests of Esculapius (400BC). The 'Art of Physic' *(sic)* or internal medicine established the aetiology of disease by applying the principles of metaphysics, that is, establishing the cause of a disease by intuitive reasoning and without any empirical foundation. For centuries, then, an illness's aetiology was fathomed by British physicians from a corpus of metaphysically-based medical knowledge founded in antiquity by the ancient Greek physicians Galen and Hippocrates. The corpus of classical and medieval medicines were based on their models of Physic. Illness was an individual experience and was understood by physicians in terms of a patient's individual *complaints* of sickness. Sickness was the result of an imbalance in an individual's humours. Galen popularised the belief that the human constitution was comprised of four humours: blood, phlegm, and black and yellow bile. Normal health depended on a balance of these humours commensurate with the individual's age and personality, while all illness was caused by one single disease which created their imbalance. Humoural pathology – which was popular in Britain until well into the nineteenth century – like all systems of physic, was monistic, that is, all illness was regarded to have resulted from one underlying pathological state and could be cured by a single method of therapy. These included the traditional depleting procedures of blood-letting, purging, blistering, cold affusions, accompanied by an assortment of homeopathic drugs. Excrementory humours aside, the pre-scientific period was also one of excrementory therapeutics, with the London Pharmacopoeia of 1618 listing the therapeutic qualities of perspiration and saliva as well as wood lice![6]

Humouralism was based on a metaphysical understanding of pathological principles. That is, disease was understood as a pathological state by applying intuitive reasoning when comparing those who were in good health with those afflicted by ill-health. Disease therefore resided in the body but its aetiology was not localised to a particular organ. Disease was also considered a natural, individual and inevitable phenomenon which should be allowed to run its course with minimal intervention by physicians. Indeed in eighteenth-century France the home was considered the natural place for those suffering from disease. Physicians themselves were therefore disinclined to intervene in its progress, preferring instead to adhere to the dictate, 'Observe the sick, assist nature without violating and wait, admitting in all modesty that much knowledge is still lacking.'[7]

The same metaphysical method which underlined humoural pathology was used to conceptualise the principles which governed the living body. Life was perceived as a series of functions which, it was reasoned, existed in order to keep death at bay. However, prior to the late eighteenth century, several attempts were made to break with the metaphysical method on which these pathological principles were established. Among the most notable of these took place at the University of Leiden in the Netherlands.[8]

Boerhaave, who taught medicine at the University from 1701 to 1738 was among the first to systematically challenge the existing metaphysical notions of Life and agitated for the replacement of 'physic' as an art (and by implication susceptible to subjective interpretation) with that of a science. Rejecting the methodology of speculative metaphysics on the premise that no pathology based on monistic principles could adequately explain the compositional elements of Life, Boerhaave formulated a system of physic which attempted to describe Life as an entity, analytically separable from its manifest effect in the living organism. If these elements were to be grasped, Boerhaave maintained, medicine would have to adopt an eclectic approach based on mechanistic principles: 'Let anatomy faithfully describe the parts and structure of the body; let mechanicians apply their particular science to the solids; let hydrostatics, their action as they move through the given canals; and lastly, let the chemist add to all of these . . . and then . . . we shall have a complete account of medical physiology.'[9]

This new eclectic medicine required the traditional, purely theoretical, abstract and dogmatic approaches to medical therapy with its orthodox speculative methodology, to be abandoned. Boerhaave was concerned instead with empirical *facts*. The search for facts was undoubtedly the main thing. Medicine should be advanced by 'just reasoning', but this should be indulged in only with great caution. Mere conjectures should be rejected, retaining only what results from observation or what follows of consequence. When, therefore, a problem presents itself, not accountable for but under hypothesis, we should restrain our judgement and leave doubts to be resolved by posterity, when they have obtained light enough from experiments which have escaped us. By this means physic 'tis true, will be reduced to a small compass, but then it will be true, certain and always the same'.[10] But Boerhaave's appeal to empirical observation, rather than pure speculation, as the methodological basis for observing the body was ultimately founded on an abstract concept of the governing principles of Life – that is as a set of mechanical actions.

Locating the principles governing the internal organs in the living body was inseparably linked to efforts by physicians to locate the disease's organic source. Little attempt, however, was made in Britain to study or classify diseases until the mid-eighteenth century. Classical and medieval medicine was concerned with the various *conditions* of the sick individual, i.e. a combination of being too hot/cold, wet/dry, and so forth. Therefore a pathological understanding of sickness was limited to theories purporting to explain man's pathological condition in terms of either bodily fluids (humouralism) or muscle and nerve conditions (solidism). It was Haller who popularised the latter, particularly in Europe, while the influence of Dr John Gregory, professor of Medicine at Edinburgh, ensured the popularity of humouralism in Britain during the early nineteenth century. Gregory's influence in British medical thought was all pervasive. 'Gregorian Physic – free blood letting, cold affusion; brisk purging, frequent blisters, the nauseating action of tartar-emetic came to rule the medical practice for many years, in all quarters throughout the British Islands and the Colonies . . . England and Ireland, as well as Scotland, together with our colonial dependencies, were overrun by his disciplines and his doctrines.'[11] Attempts in Great Britain to establish disease as an objective, substantial entity which could be associated with a distinct pathological state was made by the celebrated English physician, Thomas Sydenham (1624–89).

Rejecting medicine's conventional metaphysical methodology whereby hypotheses regarding the nature of disease and the principles governing Life could be tested by reasoning, Sydenham proceeded to passively *observe* the disease in the body. He records: 'I have been very careful to write nothing but what was the product of faithful observation, and neither suffered myself to be deceived by idle speculation, nor having deceived others by obtruding anything upon them, but downright matter of fact.'[12]

Applying this methodology Sydenham concluded diseases constituted independent entities, separable from the body. Whereas orthodox medical opinion spoke of a single disease that explained all pathological conditions, Sydenham talked of *diseases* – analytically separable entities which could manifest themselves in different patients yet in the same form. The disease's emancipation from the body (now recognised as no more than its concrete support), allowed physicians to record the same disease in a number of patients. But doctors were unable to distinguish a pathology of phenomena (which classified diseases on the basis of observed symptoms) from a pathology of 'cures' (which classified diseases on the basis of morbid pathological lesions beneath the visible symptoms). Classifying diseases in accordance with a set of symptoms (nosology) characterised British medical practice well into the nineteenth century. Attempts to break with the established medical view of Life as comprising metaphysically established principles continued alongside nosological practices. For example William Cullen, a nineteenth-century physician, organised the body pathologically into its 'vital' and 'non-vital' parts. 'The solid parts of the body seem to be of two kinds: one whose properties are the same in the dead as in the living, and the same in the animate as in the inanimate bodies. In the last, a peculiar organisation, or addition, is supposed to take place; in opposition to which, the first are called SIMPLE SOLIDS . . . and of the others which may be called VITAL SOLIDS, being the fundemental part of the nervous system.'[13] 'Life' thus existed pathologically as a balance not of humours but of certain 'vital forces'. But explaining 'Life' in terms of vitalist forces served only to focus medical attention on the disease's effects on the nervous system where it supposedly created an imbalance.

THE CLINIC

Despite efforts to formulate a pathology on new principles governing the living body such as Cullen's 'vital forces', they remained indistinct from the old pathologies of 'humouralism' and 'solidism'. In order to break with a pathology based on metaphysical 'systems of physic' a new way of establishing the principles of Life within the body was required. During the late eighteenth century such a development occurred. A change in the role and functioning of Parisian hospitals gave rise to the possibility of the medical 'Gaze'.

Originally the concept of hospitals as places for medical treatment stood in opposition to dominant eighteenth-century political and economic thinking in France. The sick placed an unnecessary burden on society; for the sick to remain in their home cost the state nothing, but the patient, occupying a hospital bed *and* incapable of working placed a double burden on society. Hospitals that did exist, both in France and Britain, emerged primarily as homes for the poor or the desperately sick who had no family to support them. Financed by philanthropic charitable concerns and lacking any effective medical therapy, they were popularly known in France as 'Temples of Death' – a reputation clearly earned, as the following eighteenth-century account illustrates:

> The general policy of the Hotel Dieu – policy caused by lack of space – is to put as many beds as possible into one room and put four, five or six people into one bed. We have seen the dead mixed with the living there. We have seen rooms so narrow that the air stagnates and is not renewed and that the light enters only feebly and charged with vapours. We have seen convalescents together with the sick, the dying and the dead, forced to go barefoot to the bridge in summer and winter when they needed fresh air. We have seen a room for convalescents on the third floor which could be reached only via the small-pox ward. The ward for the insane is next to the one for the unfortunate post-operative patients who cannot hope for rest in this neighbourhood which is full of outcries day and night.[14]

Early nineteenth-century British hospitals too, remained the province largely of the poor and desperate, as Professor Christison of the University of Edinburgh observed in 1836: 'It is chiefly when dysentery is violent from the first, or becomes so through neglect or unsuccessful treatment, that recourse is had to a hospital by the working classes.'[15] Prior to establishing hospitals as places for teaching, observation and therapy, or 'clinics'[16] medical education and practical training was given individually, privately and at considerable expense of time and money, by elite physicians. The British attempt to establish clinics was considerably less auspicious than its development in France. In 1720, Alexander Monro, together with other former pupils of Boerhaave, established a clinic adjoining the main building of the medical faculty at the University of Edinburgh. This provided a unique opportunity for medical students to study diseases in the living patient as well as to receive systematic instruction at the patient's bedside. The patient's body then became a teaching aid which revealed through recorded observations the progress and development of diseases. However, the Edinburgh clinic was not replicated on a nationwide scale, as state-funded aid to finance a re-structuring programme was not made available.[17]

Fever hospitals which mushroomed throughout England during the period 1817–1820 'on account of the extensive spread of fever in the epidemic form among the working classes', continued to base their therapies on monistic pathologies. Fevers were categorised according to Cullen's taxonomies based on the disease's symptoms, and treatment followed the ancient practices of cold affusions and blood-letting. Only when the symptoms could be recorded statistically, by doctors freed from an exclusively therapeutic role, was the concept of a 'case' (a diseased state comprising a collection of different symptoms) possible.

British doctors, therefore, seeking the anatomo-pathological 'seat' of the disease at autopsies, were confounded. Any physiological organ which did not look 'right' could simply be reduced to the effects of death upon the body. Christison, in his account of the search for the morbid source of typhoid fever notes:

> We saw nothing then; nor for many years afterwards. It might have been overlooked during life, it could not have been missed during death. For our dissections were many, and to meet the bias of the day for finding an anatomical cause for all fevers, every important organ in the body was habitually looked to. Nevertheless, we were constantly met with want of morbid appearances anywhere, unless the slight signs of vascular congestion in various membranous textures be considered such – signs, however, which were probably nothing else than the result of the manner of death, by slow arrestment of the respiration under oppression of the brain.[18]

The inability of British medicine to perceive a 'case' was in fact part of a wider failure to 'observe' the sick. In British hospitals throughout much of the nineteenth century, the emphasis was upon *cure* and *therapeutics* as opposed to observation. Built largely from charitable donations, medical practice, tightly controlled by these philanthropists, was required to produce results. The absence of state-funded support for the development of hospitals along the lines of the clinic and the consequent absence of widespread opportunities for medical research until the late nineteenth century, reflect the low status of medicine in Britain during this period.[19]

In contrast, the restructuring of Parisian hospitals along the lines of the Leiden model during the late eighteenth century, was part of a wider post-revolutionary period restructuring of the faculties for the poor and the sick. A public health movement funded by central government was introduced, and hospitals, instead of relying on philanthropic charities for funding, became state-financed. Hospital doctors were released from the financial constraints of the patronage system and from the traditional therapeutic role – blindly preoccupied with dubious therapy – to become clinicians whose work held a greater emphasis on recording signs and symptoms in order to deal with the primary problem of diagnosis and classification of disease.

From these recordings emerged a picture of disease as a *collection* of symptoms instead of each symptom representing a specific ailment. Clinicians therefore spoke not of a pathology of symptoms but a pathology of disease; not an individual illness, but a 'case' – an endlessly reproducible series of signs and symptoms which indicated a single disease. Locating the pathological source or seat of the disease within the body however required doctors to *decipher* the manifest, visible symptoms as indicators of the disease's morbid pathological seat which lay within the recesses of the body. Shyrock captures this point in illustrating the case of tuberculosis. 'One man working at the bedside, describes a symptom complex involving coughing and fever, known as consumption; another man, at his dissecting table, noted in the lungs the small nodules known as tubercles. The symptomatic conception of consumption could be made more specific and meaningful only when it was associated with the tubercles discovered by the pathologist.'[20] But to develop a morbid pathology, i.e. locating the seat of a disease within the body's organs, required a new understanding of the principles which governed the living body that did not merely impute their existence by reasoning but could be understood empirically. This is because lesions discovered in the diseased body after death could still be conceptualised as merely accompanying death, and not contributing to its cause.

The celebrated nineteenth-century French physiologist, Xaviar Bichat, established a pathology which rejected the earlier vitalist notions. Disease resided not in the vital organs, creating in turn a nervous imbalance, but in the tissues which constitute these vital organs. These tissues, Bichat maintained, 'are linked together only by direct relations of organisation with the neighbouring parts'.[21] Death was conceptualised as resulting from a break in this link but it might not immediately extinguish life. 'Death is . . . multiple and dispersed in time: it is not that absolute, privileged point at which time stops, and moves back; like disease itself, it has a teeming presence that analysis may divide into time and space, gradually, here and there, each of the knots breaks until organic life ceases.'[22]

Physicians then, could examine the living disease in the corpse because the death of the host no longer immediately rendered the disease's pathological morbid lesions invisible to the enquiring eye of the clinician. But a reading of the symptoms with intent to intervene in the course of the disease was still beyond the scope of medical practice because Life continued to be discussed as an effect which, it was speculated, existed only as a *function* produced by the organisation of the organs within the body. But the conditions governing this function did not yet exist and until these conditions were empirically established doctors remained unable to establish Life as an experimentally materialisable phenomenon.

MATERIALISING LIFE WITHIN THE LABORATORY

The new perception of life as a materialisable phenomenon within the body was possible from new experimental techniques of medical research. Working in a laboratory where experiments were conducted within controlled conditions Magendie, a nineteenth-century physiologist and Professor of Medicine at the University of Paris, accomplished a break with the orthodox understanding of the governing principles of Life. Magendie maintained Life was not that which resulted from the sum of the functions of the organs, but was simply the regulating activity of the organs.

However it was not Magendie who applied this principle to medical research, but his pupil, the equally eminent physiologist Claude Bernard. Bernard spoke of Life, not speculatively – as an undifferentiated property of the constituent elements making up the pathological organ's tissues – but as a materialisable object conceptualised as a mechanism which is maintained only by the balance of functional activities of what he termed the histological units: the minute structure of the tissues. In Bernard's wake, by the late nineteenth century, it was possible for physicians to talk of the 'life' of a cell or the 'life' of an organ, as distinct from the holistic organic Life of the body. This new formulation of Life (and Death) was made explicit in Bernard's discussion on the effects of carbon monoxide poisoning; 'death came through death of the molecules of blood, or in other words by stopping their exercise of a physiological property essential to life'.[23] The gas displaces the oxygen in the blood cells thereby destroying them. This in turn sets off a chain reaction. Tissues relying on these cells for their supply of oxygen are starved and begin to die. As more and more tissue dies the whole organism eventually expires.

Bernard had replaced the enigmatic notion of Life with an experimentally observable one defined in terms of the conditions governing its existence. These conditions or laws were revealed experimentally. One such law, for example, governed organic self-regulation – the principle wherein the disease's progress could be observed in living tissue and the tissue experimented upon to establish the disease's pathological cause. 'Thanks to their organic self-regulation we can also detach living tissues; and by means of artificial circulation or otherwise we can place them in conditions where we can better study their characteristics.'[24]

Once the laws governing the disease's conditions of existence had been established, it was possible for doctors to directly intervene in the disease's progress. Disease was no longer a substantial entity which existed independently from the body but was a malfunction in one of the conditions of existence of living organisms. The physiological (normal) and the pathological (diseased) state are therefore governed by the same law. Diseases are therefore defined in the same terms as physiological phenomena under normal conditions: 'Diseases at bottom are only physiological phenomena in new conditions still to be determined; toxic and medicinal action . . . come back to simple physiological changes in properties of the histological units of our tissues.'[25]

The Rolleston Report defined addiction as a disease in just such terms in 1926. The addicted state was considered basically as Life under abnormal conditions whereby the toxic action of the opiate produced changes in the conditions of normal physiological functioning (the basis of pharmacological dependence). However medicinal action (in the form of maintenance prescriptions of opiates) was designed to retain these altered conditions of physiological functioning on the understanding that opiate-induced pathological changes had become a feature of the physiological law governing normal functioning. The Report thus stated that in certain circumstances addiction

> must be regarded as a disease and not as a mere form of vicious indulgence. In other words, the drug is taken in such cases not

for the purpose of obtaining positive pleasure but in order to relieve a morbid and powerful craving. The actual need for the drug in extreme cases is so great that, if it is not administered, great physical distress, culminating in actual collapse and even death, may result, unless special precautions are taken such as can only be carried out under close medical supervision, and with careful nursing.[26]

POSTSCRIPT

The Rolleston Report clearly marked a new episode in the history of responses to drug use. It made provisions for doctors to legitimately treat addicts with opiate drugs. It also affirmed the doctors' rights to professional self-regulation. Doctors who were authorised to possess and prescribe opiates would be accountable to a Medical Tribunal and not be subject to regulation by the State.[27]

However the Home Office's acceptance of the Rolleston Report's recommendations did not signal a complete shift in thinking to addiction as a medical rather than a moral issue. In 1937 Dr E.W.Adams, a member of the Rolleston Committee, set out the medical opinion on habitual drug use in his book *Drug Addiction*, which he dedicated to the Committee's chairman, Humphrey Rolleston, and which contained chapters on epidemiology, diagnosis and prognosis. Under aetiology, he wrote, 'The underlying cause is not, in many instances, mere viciousness and, even where that is so, the more enlightened opinion of recent years regards the drug habit, however acquired, not as a crime to be punished but as a disease to be treated', but adds, 'Though addiction, when fully established, ought to be regarded and treated as a disease . . . it is certain that it may originate in vice.' And though provisions were made for medically defined treatment of addiction the report also retained provisions for penal legislation – with possession of dangerous drugs within the schedules of the Dangerous Drugs Acts (1920, 1923) without a prescription – still the subject of criminal proceedings.[28]

The importance of the report in the history of responses to drug addiction should not be understated. Its recommendations contained the blueprint for what became known abroad (especially in the USA) as a distinctive 'British approach' in which doctors rather than policemen were to deal with drug addicts, and contrasted starkly with efforts in the United States during the same period to criminalise addiction. Many British observers have since claimed that there was no such distinct approach, 'only loose guidelines about treatment.'[29] Notwithstanding their claims, the Rolleston Report did signpost a new era in which medicine could, for the first time in its involvement with drug addiction, offer the possibility of exclusively treating the addict's body.

9 Conclusion

Adams[1] argues that after De Quincey the next chapter in the history of drug use opens with two important events: the isolation of morphine and the invention of the hypodermic syringe. Recently Berridge and Edwards[2] and Parssinen[3] have concurred on the significance of these developments as milestones in the development of responses to addiction in this country. Undoubtedly changes in the type of opiate consumed and mode of its administration played their part in sharpening the focus of public attention on the phenomenon of opiate dependence. The growing late nineteenth-century trend for injected morphine, with its strikingly obvious attendant psycho-pharmacological effects on the addict compared against the effects of laudanum drinking, also served to heighten public concern.

Forms of social control have also played a role in shaping nineteenth-century judgements on opium consumption. In this respect one cannot dismiss, for example, the significance of the rationalisation of the human body as a work tool, and the instilling of industrial work discipline, which took place with the development of industrial capitalism. These practices based on class relations were clearly of importance in promoting notions of economically-determined behaviour as 'rational' and thereby taking precedence over culturally determined 'irrational' behaviour such as the 'opium habit'. But neither factor adequately explains how the dramatic changes in the ways addiction could be talked about since the nineteenth century were possible. Conventional histories of responses to opium dependence begin from what is already known about nineteenth-century moral reformists and the development of medical specialisms. Institutionalised responses to opium dependence then become arranged to form a linear progression which reflects the accumulation of rational thought. Berridge and Edwards' thesis encapsulates this approach. The development of concern over opium use is connected with some form of veiled social control by the public health movement and the political machinations of the medical and pharmaceutical professions, which becomes sharply focused with the 'discovery' of morphine and an increasing propensity for administering it hypodermically.

Even Parssinen, who argues that Berridge and Edwards' account of the role of social control 'stretches a thinly worn phrase well past its breaking point,'[4] does not escape the implications of conventional historicism. In his reworking of the historical material on responses to opium dependence, Parssinen openly acknowledges his allegiance to a conventional historical approach, viz.: 'the historian is a detective. He must locate the body, then find out whodunnit and why'.[5]

Such approaches to the development of responses to drugs are underscored by a view of the past which may be analogous to a long corridor on which are hung pictures of great 'discoveries' and events of the past. At the far end of the corridor are placed pictures depicting the discovery of the wheel. Further along the corridor, and further on in time, are pictures showing the discovery of planetary motion, electricity, penicillin and so forth. Conventional historians of opium dependence would hang pictures of the first moral and medical responses along these corridors – arranging them as causally discovered facts about the nature of opium dependence so they form a time-scale which reflects the steady but gradual accumulation of knowledge. Conventionally then, historians have looked back to the past in order to locate the beginnings of moralists' and medical specialists' statements or distinctive language on opium dependence.

In contrast to these conventional histories I have attempted to sketch the outline of a different history of responses – an account which, methodologically at least, owes much to the writings of the iconoclast Michel Foucault, in particular *The Archaeology of Knowledge*[6] and *Discipline and Punish.*[7] In applying this methodology to the development of responses to opiate addiction, I have attempted not to survey the history of moral or medical responses as pre-given unities: to locate a specific point in time when opium dependence first became discovered as an issue of moral or medical concern. Nor have I wished to establish an understanding of opium dependence as a typically representative moral or medical view. The initial categorisation of opium dependence, based on an analysis of the moral status of the addict, and latterly as a medically defined disease is therefore not held out as representing an achievement of scientific rationality. These categories, I have argued, are not 'discovered' purposively, following the intense activities of enquiring minds.

Moralists did not simply turn their attention to opium dependence in order to 'see' beneath the level of appearances and peer at the addict's moral faculty. Similarly, medically-qualified addiction specialists could not simply cast their trained eye over the addict's body to suddenly discover within it a pathological disease. Rather, both categories existed fundamentally as social products of different processes that have little direct relevance to the development of the nineteenth-century moral reformist movement or to the medical profession's newly discovered political muscle following its consolidated reorganisation.

Instead of asking when the first distinctive moral or medical statements on addiction emerged, I have tried to describe the social relations which made possible these descriptions and the way in which they could be taken seriously. In doing so I have been guided to a wide range of source material, some whose connection with opium use are at times tentative and some which are occasionally obscure. These have lead me to alter the timescale for the first responses to addiction. Following De Quincey's revelations of 1822, the next chapter in the history of responses to addiction is not a medical one – set by the trend for hypodermic injections of morphine – but a moral one following the establishment of the SSOT in the early 1870s. Unlike conventional accounts I have argued that a definitely medical response did not follow hard on the heels of a newly established group of medical specialists on addiction during the 1880s, but instead followed changes in the way doctors understood the functioning of their patients' bodies. The application of this new understanding to a state of addiction is not evidenced until the 1920s when the Rolleston Committee's deliberations were reported.

The idea that there might be cases of addicts who having contracted the habit showed no 'noticeable moral, mental or physical deterioration . . . [who] are in no real sense degenerate' and who may be authorised to continue taking the drug for the rest of their lives was reiterated by Adams in 1937.[8] For the first time since widespread concern began to be expressed about drug addiction during the 1870s, it was possible for the charge of individual responsibility for one's addiction to be suspended, and this became increasingly likely as the disease model of addiction gained currency among doctors and policy-makers alike. Some features of drug policy in the 1920s currently remain but doctors no longer occupy a key position in dealing with addiction. As we move into the final decades of the twentieth century, prohibitionist policies such as the seizure of illegal opiate imports and an increase in successful prosecutions for drug trafficking are increasingly favoured against medical treatment facilities for addicts which have produced a poor return. Possibly we are witnessing another change in the conception of addiction similar in scope at least to that which took place over sixty years ago. Proposals to dispense free needles to addicts as a measure to contain the spread of AIDS apparently appear to condone the 'lesser' evil of opiates in an attempt to control an even greater one. If this is the case, perhaps then we should be looking beyond the medical profession and the state for our evidence?

Notes and References

Introduction

1. J. Thompson, *Medical Times*, 1840; no.1, pp.162 – 3.
2. E. Levinstein *Morbid Cravings for Morphia*, C. Harrier (London: Smith, Elder & co. 1878) pp.109 – 18.
3. Interim Report of the Canadian Government Commission of Enquiry: *Non-Medical Use of Drugs* (Harmondsworth: Penguin 1971).
4. J. Jaffe and W. Martin, Narcotic Analgesics and Antagonists', *The Pharmacological Basis of Therapeutics*, ed. L. S. Goddman and A. Gilman, 5th edition (New York: Macmillan, 1975).
5. T. Sydenham 1680 quoted in G. V. Stimson and E. Oppenheimer, *Heroin Addiction Treatment and Control in Britain* (London and New York: Tavistock 1982) p.13.
6. Quoted in E.W.Adams, *Drug Addiction* (London: Oxford University Press, 1937) p.1.

1 Opium and the British

1. Quoted in E. W. Adams, *Drug Addiction* (London: Oxford University Press, 1937).
2. V. Berridge and N. Lawson, 'Opiate use and legislative control: a nineteenth century case study', *Social Science and Medicine* 1979; 13a: pp.351 – 63, p.353.
3. V. Berridge, 'Working class opium eating in the nineteenth century: establishing the facts', *British Journal of Addiction* 1978; 73; pp.363 – 74, p.363.
4. V. Berridge and G. Edwards, *Opium and the People* (London: Allen Lane, 1981) p.25.
5. V. Berridge B. J. A., 1978; 73: pp.363 – 74, p.368.
6. V. Berridge, 'Victorian Opium Eating: Responses to Opiate Use in Nineteenth-Century England', *Victorian Studies* 1978; 21, No.4: pp.437 – 61, p.441.
7. J. Pereira, *The Elements of Materia Medica and Therapeutics*, Vol.II (Philadelphia: Lea & Blanchard, 1843) p.703.
8. Berridge and Edwards, *Opium and the People* p.25.
9. V. Berridge, 'Our own opium: Cultivation of the opium poppy in Britain, 1740 – 1823', *British Journal of Addiction* 1977; 72; pp.90 – 94.
10. Berridge and Edwards, *Opium and the People*, p.16.
11. T. De Quincey, *Confessions of an English Opium Eater* (London: J. H. Dent 1972) p.xiii.
12. Quoted in *The Dictionary of Biographical Quotation of British and American Subjects*, eds. J.Wintle and R.Kenin (London: Routledge & Kegan Paul, 1978).

13. E. Schnider, *Coleridge, Opium and Kubla Khan.* (University of Chicago Press, 1953).
14. A. Hayter, *Opium and the Romantic Imagination* (London: Faber & Faber, 1968).
15. Berridge and Edwards, *Opium and the People*, p.85.
16. Ibid, p.259.
17. Ibid.
18. V. Berridge B.J.A. 1978; 73; p.368.
19. T. De Quincey, Quoted in Berridge and Edwards *Opium and the People*, p.105.
20. Parliamentary Paper 'Report from the Select Committee on Inquiry into Drunkenness, No.VIII', 1834 p.325.
21. Parliamentary Paper, Factory Inquiry Commission: Supplementary Report of the Central Board, No.XIX, 1834 pp.538 – 9.
22. Parliamentary Papers, Report from the Select Committee on Inquiry into Drunkenness, 1834, p.325.
23. T. M. Parssinen, Essay Review of Berridge and Edwards *Opium and the People, Medical History,* 1982 pp.458 – 462.
24. Parliamentary Paper, Report of the Commissioners for Inquiring into the State of Large Towns and Populous Districts: XVIII, 1844.
25. 'Medicus', 'Teetotalism and Opium Taking', *Lancet* 1851, p.694.

2 The Indo-Chinese Opium Wars

1. 'A Short History of a Great Wrong', Pamphlet issued in connection with the 'United Christian Appeal for the Ending of the Indo-Chinese Opium Traffic' under the Auspices of the Representative Board of the London Anti-Opium Societies. See *Braithwaite Collection* Anti-opium tracts and resolutions 1850–1914/15, Friends House Library, Euston Rd, London NW1.
2. Ibid
3. SSOT pamphlet, *The Opium Trade with China* (London: Dyer Brothers, 1880) p.5.
4. 'A Short History of a Great Wrong', SSOT pamphlet.
5. 'England and the Opium Trade', SSOT pamphlet p.6.
6. 'A Short History of a Great Wrong', SSOT pamphlet.

3 The Anti-Opium Crusade

1. J. Rowntree, *The Imperial Drug Trade* (London: Methuen, 1905) p.268.
2. W. T. Wu, *The Chinese Opium Question in British Opinion and Action* (New York: Academy Press, 1928).
3. D. E. Owen, *British Opium Policy in China and India* (New Haven: Yale University Press, 1934).
4. P. Lowes, *The Genesis of International Narcotics Control* (Geneva: Librarie Droz, 1966).
5. J. B. Brown, 'Politics of the Poppy: The Society for the Suppression of the Opium Trade 1874–1916', *Journal of Contemporary History,* 1973; no.3, vol.8, pp.97 – 111.

6. B. Johnson, 'Righteousness Before Revenue: The Forgotten Crusade Against the Indo-Chinese Opium Trade', *Journal of Drug Issues*, 1975; 5; pp.304 – 26.
7. *Braithwaite Collection*, Society of Friends M5. vol.207, p.9.
8. London Yearly Meeting, 1858; Extracts of Minutes and Proceedings, Appendix B, p.54.
9. Johnson, J. D. I., 1975, p.305.
10. See *Friend of China*, vol.IV, August 1880, no.6, p.141.
11. Reports of the SSOT's activities were also to be found in Anti-Opium News, a mid-monthly supplement to the *Sentinel* which ran from March 1891 until June 1893 – published by the Association for the Improvement of Public Morals.
12. See Johnson J. D. I. 1975 p.311.
13. The Shanghai convention was inaugurated at the instigation of the Americans on 1 February 1909. It was concerned initially with the Indian Opium trade with China, though the focus did widen from control of opiates exported to the Far East, to control of domestic use in the West. It was followed by further international conventions in 1911–12, 1913 and 1914, at the Hague.

4 Constructing Addiction as a Moral Failing

1. Rev G. John, Plain Questions and Straightforward Answers about the Opium Trade', *Braithwaite Collection*
2. *Friend of China*, vol.VI, no.4, April 1883, p.106.
3. *Friend of China*, vol.X, no.8, April 1888.
4. *Friend of China*, vol.X. no.8, April 1881, p.207.
5. Rev. G. John, *Braithwaite Collection* 'Plain Questions' p.21.
6. *Friend of China*, vol.IV, no.9, February 1881, p.235.
7. Letter from J. W. Pease to Rt Hon Viscount Cross 1892 British Museum ref x529/1031.
8. A. S. Dyer in *'Suffering for the Truth'* by M. Gregory 1894 (pamphlet) Braithwate Collection
9. *Friend of China*, December 1892, pp.266 – 68.
10. Rev G. John, *Braithwaite Collection.*
11. 'A Great Moral Wrong', *Braithwaite Collection*, p.6.
12. *Friend of China*, vol.XV, no.4 May 1895, Supplement: Royal Commission on Opium: Minutes of Dissent Q8805 and Q15146.

5 Opium and the Quakers

1. For the procedure by which Quaker membership has historically been conferred see R.Vann, *The Social Development of English Quakerism 1655–1755* (Massachusetts: Harvard University Press, 1969) p.144.
2. *Friend of China*, vol.X, no.8 April 1888, p.214.
3. *Christian Doctrine of the Society of Friends*, Friends Tract Association, 1904, p.100.
4. London Yearly Meeting of Friends, Extracts from Minutes and Proceedings, 1881, p.1.

5. E. Isichei, *Victorian Quakers* (London: Oxford University Press, 1970).
6. London Yearly Meeting of Friends, Extract from Minutes and Proceedings, 1857, p.27.
7. R. Howard, *The Church of England and other Religious Communions* (London: Keegan, Paul, Trench, 1885).
8. See M. Kirby, *Men of Business and Politics* (London: Allen & Unwin, 1984).
9. London Yearly Meeting of Friends, Extracts from Minutes and Proceedings, 1834 p.44.
10. Anon, *The Physiology of the Sects* (London: Samuel Tinsley, 1874) p.147.
11. R. Howard, *The Church of England* p.70.
12. L. Stephen and S. Lee (eds) *Dictionary of National Biography* No.44 (London: Oxford University Press) p.179.
13. J. Evans, *A Sketch of the Denominations of the Christian World* (London: Baldwin, Cradock & Joy 1827).
14. E. Isichei, *Victorian Quakers*, p.87.
15. Some 20 000 copies of an anti-opium tract, 'An Appeal to our Countrymen', were published and distributed by the Society of Friends in 1881. See Extracts of the London Yearly Meeting, 1881 p.25.
16. Extract from the Minutes and Proceedings of the Yearly Meeting of Friends, 1859, Appendix B p.54, Note also: Sub-Committees of these Meetings for Suffering which were subsequently formed, and which were concerned directly with the anti-opium trafficking campaign included the Home Office Committee, established in 1882, and the Committee of the Friends' Foreign Mission Association, established in 1868. Both exercised considerable independent power despite being technically subordinate to the Yearly Meeting.
17. Friends of the Opium Question, *Friend of China* 1880, vol.IV, no.3; pp.73–4.
18. London Yearly Meeting of Friends, Extracts from Minutes and Proceedings, 1880, p.23.

6 Forming the Moral Pathological Model as an Object

1. Berridge and Edwards p.53.
2. For examples of how the literary circles of the early nineteenth century saw the issue of addiction as one of humour see: 'Noctes Ambrosianae', *Blackwood's Edinburgh Magazine*, 1823, 14: pp.485–6; and 'A recent confession of an opium eater', ibid, 1856, 80; pp.629–39.
3. See *Medical Intelligencer*, no.3, 1822, pp.116–8.
4. *Confessions of an English Opium Eater,* reviewed in *The British Review and London Critical Journal*, 1822, 20; pp.474–88.
5. *Friend of China*, vol.XII, no.1, January 1891, p.18.
6. *Friend of China*, vol.XIII, no.3, May 1892.
7. *The Confessions of Aleister Crowley,* Symonds and Grant (eds) (London: Jonathan Cape, 1969) p.35.
8. Ibid, p.486.
9. Ibid, p.486.
10. Ibid, p.400.
11. Ibid, p.722.

12. *Friend of China*, vol.XI no.5, January 1890
13. *Friend of China*, vol.I. no.4, October 1876, p.209.
14. *Friend of China*, vol.VI, no.9, September 1883, pp.239–41.
15. *Friend of China* Supplement to vol.XIII, no.4, July 1892, 'The Medical Aspects of the Opium Question', reported, 'It may be true that we cannot point to any definitive pathological conditions continually associated with the opium habit' (p.11).
16. *Friend of China*, vol.II, No.8 March 1877.
17. *Friend of China*, vol.XVII, no.I January 1897. Similar examples can be drawn from many issues of *Friend of China*, in particular see vol.XIII, no.4; vol.XXIII, no.3; vol.II, no.8.
18. *Friend of China*, vol.XIII, no.1, January 1892, p.11.
19. *Friend of China*, vol.XIII, no.4, July 1892.
20. *Friend of China*, vol.IX, no.2, June 1886, p.34.
21. *Friend of China*, vol.X, no.8, April 1888, p.214.
22. *Friend of China*, vol.XI, no.6, April 1890.
23. Ibid.
24. *Friend of China*, vol.XVII, no.2, April 1897.
25. *Friend of China*, vol.XVIII, no.7, December 1892 lists the General Secretary of the Baptist Missionary Society and a representative of the Union Chapel, Manchester, as council members.
26. *Friend of China*, vol.XVIII, no.3, July 1891.

7 From Moral Weakness to Pathological Disease

1. B. Johnson, J. D. I., 1975.
2. H. Becker, *The Outsider* (New York: Free Press, 1963) pp.147–8.
3. M. Ward, *Facts establishing the Efficacy of the Opium Friction* (London: Wheeler 1809) p.55.
4. T. C. Allbutt, 'On the Abuse of Hypodermic Injections of Morphia, '*The Practitioner*, 1870; 5: pp.329–330.
5. E. Levinstein *Morbid Cravings for Morphine* p.3.
6. Ibid, p.7.
7. *Proceedings of the Society for the Study and Cure of Inebriety*, no.1, July 1884 p.1.
8. A. Carpenter, 'The meeting place of vice and disease in the inebriate', *Proceedings*, 1887, p.20.
9. N. Kerr, *Inebriety or Narcomania; its etiology, pathology, treatment and jurisprudence*, 3rd edition (London: H. K. Lewis, 1894) p.6.
10. Ibid, p.10.
11. Ibid, p.117.
12. Ibid, pp.211–2.
13. Ibid, p.298.
14. O. Jennings, *The Re-Education of Self-Control in the Treatment of the Morphia Habit* (London: Bailliere, Tindall & Cox, 1909) p.5.
15. Ibid, p.29.
16. Ibid, p.19.
17. Ibid, p.483.
18. T. D. Crothers, *Morphinism and Narcomania from other Drugs* (London: W. B. Saunders, 1902) p.42.

19. S. Sharkey, 'Morphinomania', *Nineteenth Century*, 1887, no.22; pp.335–42.
20. H. Sainsbury, *Drugs and the Drug Habit* (London: Methuen, 1909) p.223.
21. The idea of a 'disease of the will' belonged initially to the eighteenth-century physician Benjamin Rush who first coined the term to describe the condition of alcoholism, 'The use of strong drink is at first the effect of free agency. From habit it takes place from necessity.' See M. Keller, 'On loss of control phenomenon in alcoholism', *British Journal of Addiction*, 1972, (67), pp.153–66.
22. V. Berridge, 'War Conditions and Narcotic Control: The Passing of Defence of the Realm Act Regulation 40B', *Journal of Social Policy*, 1978, vol.7, part 3; pp.285 – 304.
23. V. Berridge, 'Professionalisation and Narcotics: The Medical and Pharmaceutical Professions and British Narcotic Use', *Psychological Medicine*, 1978; no.8; pp.361-72.
24. D. F. Musto, *The American Disease: Origins of Narcotic Control* (New Haven and London: Yale University Press, 1973).
25. Report of the Departmental Committee on Morphine and Heroin Addiction (London: HMSO, 1926) p.2.
26. Ibid, p.9.
27. Ibid, p.18.
28. G. V. Stimson and E. Oppenheimer, *Heroin Addiction: Treatment and Control in Britain* (London: Tavistock, 1982).
29. Quoted by G. Edwards, 'Opium and After' *Lancet*, 16 February, 1981.
30. T. D. Crothers, *Morphinism and Narcomania*, p.141.

8 Pathology and the Medical Model

1. M. J. Peterson, *The Medical Profession in Mid-Victorian Britain* (London: University of California Press 1978).
2. Evidence of apothecaries as the only source of medical care for the working class and the poor is to be found in literature of the day. See M. F. Brightfield, 'The Medical Profession in Victorian England as depicted in the novels of the period 1840–1870', *Bulletin of the History of Medicine*, 1961, vol.35 pp.238 – 56. Cope (in Peterson, 1978) also notes that until 1815 apothecaries and druggists represented roughly three quarters of the estimated total of all medical practitioners.
3. J. R. Reynolds, 'On the Relation of Practical Medicine to Philosophic Method and Popular Opinion', Address before the North London Medical Society, 1858, p.19.
4. See for example 'Observations on Colds, Fevers, Disease of the Liver and other Disorders with directions for treating them', D.Johnson (London: Longman), Hurst *et al.* 1823, *The Express or Every Man His Own Doctor*, (Gainsborough: Arundel and Son, 1823), *The Family Surgeon and Physician or Every Man His Own Doctor*, R. Boyce (Hull: M. Turner & Co. 1824).
5. M. Foucault, *The Birth of the Clinic: An Archaeology of Medical Perception* (London: Tavistock, 1973).
6. R. H. Shryock, *The Development of Modern Medicine* (London: Victor Gollancz, 1948) p.26.
7. Lanthenas quoted in M.Foucault, *The Birth of the Clinic: An Archaeology of Medical Perception* (London: Tavistock, 1973) p.17.

8. For further information on the influence of the Leyden School see Guthrie, 'The Influence of the Leyden School on Scottish Medicine', *Medical History*, 1959; vol.3; pp.108 – 22.
9. J. Thompson, *The Work of William Cullen, vol.1* (London: W. Blackwood 1827) p.213.
10. Boerhaave quoted in R. H. Shryock, *Development of Modern Medicine*, p.65.
11. Christisons (eds), *The Life of Sir Robert Christison, Bart,* Vol.I (London: William Blackwood, 1836) p.79.
12. T. Sydenham quoted in *Dictionary of National Bibliography*, no.55 (London: Sidney Lee (ed), Lee Smith Elder & Co. 1891) p.250.
13. J. Thompson, *The Work of William Cullen*, p.10.
14. I. Waddington, 'The Role of the Hospital in the Development of Modern Medicine', *Sociology*, 1973; vol.7; no.2, pp.211 – 24, p.216.
15. Christisons(eds), *Life of Sir Robt. Christison*, p.378.
16. The term 'Clinic' is taken from M. Foucault, *Birth of the Clinic.*
17. I. Waddington *Sociology*, 1973, notes piecemeal attempts in early nineteenth-century London, Oxford and Cambridge to organise hospitals along the lines of the clinic but these were not replicated on a nationwide scale.
18. Christisons(eds), *Life of Sir Robert Christison*, p.140.
19. Public Health movements had little faith in the medicine of the day. See *Lancet*, 30 September 1848 (p.383) and 16 December 1848 (p.673). One hundred years later the situation had changed little. No physician was appointed to the first National Health Board when it was set up in 1948. (Shyrock, *Development of Modern Medicine*).
20. Ibid, p.62.
21. Bichat quoted in Foucault, *Birth of the Clinic*, p.127.
22. Ibid, p.142. Bichat was influenced by a group of French intellectuals known as the Ideologues. This group were particularly interested in the implications of philosophic empiricism for medicine. Their view that all concepts originated in sensations – that the mind is at first a blank page – naturally lent itself to an emphasis upon the careful observation of phenomena and an avoidance of speculative hypotheses. It was the Ideologues' consequent interest in localised pathology that provided Bichat's work with its point of departure.
23. C. Bernard, *Introduction a l'etude de la medicine experimentale* (1867) translated as *An Introduction to the Study of Experimental Medicine* (New York: Dover Books, 1957) p.161.
24. Ibid, p.98.
25. Ibid, p.198.
26. Report of the Departmental Committee on Morphine and Heroin Addiction, 1926, p.11.
27. Ibid, p.24.
28. The case for penal legislation to control drugs is elaborated further in V. Berridge, 'War Conditions and Narcotic Control: The Passing of Defence of the Realm Act Regulation 40B', *Journal of Social Policy*, 1978; part 3, vol.7; pp.285 – 304.
29. C. Smart, 'Social Policy and Drug Dependence: A Historical Case Study', *Drug and Alcohol Dependence* 1985; 16, pp.169 – 80.

9 Conclusion

1. E. W. Adams, *Drug Addiction*.
2. Berridge and Edwards *Opium and the People*.
3. T. M. Parssinen, *Secret Passions, Secret Remedies: Narcotic Drugs in British Society 1820–1930* (Manchester University Press; 1983).
4. T. M. Parssinen Essay Review of Berridge and Edwards, *Opium and the People*, in *Medical History*, 1982, pp.458 – 462, p.459.
5. T. M. Parssinen, *Secret Passions*, p.xi.
6. M. Foucault, *The Archaeology of Knowledge*, trans. A. M. Sheridan (London: Tavistock, 1974).
7. M. Foucault, *Discipline and Punish: The Birth of the Prison* (London: Allen Lane, 1977).
8. E. W. Adams, *Drug Addiction*, p.73.

Index